World Health Organization

The series *International Histological Classification of Tumours* consists of the following volumes. Each of these volumes – apart from volumes 1 and 2, which have already been revised – will appear in a revised edition within the next few years. Volumes of the current editions can be ordered through WHO, Distribution and Sales, Avenue Appia, CH-1211 Geneva 27.

1. Histological typing of lung tumours (1967, second edition 1981)
2. Histological typing of breast tumours (1968, second edition 1981)
3. Histological typing of soft tissue tumours (1969)
4. Histological typing of oral and oropharyngeal tumours (1971)
6. Histological typing of bone tumours (1972)
8. Cytology of the female genital tract (1973)
9. Histological typing of ovarian tumours (1973)
10. Histological typing of urinary bladder tumours (1973)
12. Histological typing of skin tumours (1974)
13. Histological typing of female genital tract tumours (1975)
14. Histological and cytological typing of neoplastic diseases of haematopoietic and lymphoid tissues (1976)
16. Histological typing of testis tumours (1977)
17. Cytology of non-gynaecological sites (1977)
20. Histological typing of tumours of the liver, biliary tract and pancreas (1978)
22. Histological typing of prostate tumours (1980)
23. Histological typing of endocrine tumours (1980)
24. Histological typing of tumours of the eye and its adnexa (1980)
25. Histological typing of kidney tumours (1981)

A coded compendium of the International Histological Classification of Tumours (1978).

The following volumes have already appeared in a revised edition with Springer Verlag:
Histological Typing of Thyroid Tumours, 2nd edn. Hedinger/Williams/Sobin (1988)
Histological Typing of Intestinal Tumours, 2nd edn. Jass/Sobin (1989)
Histological Typing of Oesophageal and Gastric Tumours, 2nd edn. Watanabe/Jass/Sobin (1990)
Histological Typing of Tumours of the Gallbladder and Extrahepatic Bile Ducts, 2nd edn. Albores-Saavedra/Henson/Sobin (1990)
Histological Typing of Tumours of the Upper Respiratory Tract and Ear, 2nd edn. Shanmugaratnam/Sobin (1991)
Histological Typing of Salivary Gland Tumours, 2nd edn. Seifert (1991)
Histological Typing of Odontogenic Tumours, 2nd edn. Kramer/Pindborg/Shear (1992)
Histological Typing of Tumours of the Central Nervous System, 2nd edn. Kleihues/Burger/Scheithauer (1993)

Histological Typing of Tumours of the Central Nervous System

P. Kleihues, P.C. Burger, and B.W. Scheithauer

In Collaboration with L. H. Sobin and Pathologists in 14 Countries

Second Edition

With 106 Figures

Springer-Verlag
Berlin Heidelberg New York
London Paris Tokyo
Hong Kong Barcelona
Budapest

P. Kleihues
Institute of Neuropathology, University Hospital
CH-8091 Zurich, Switzerland

P. C. Burger
Department of Pathology, The Johns Hopkins University
Baltimore, Maryland 21287, USA

B. W. Scheithauer
Department of Laboratory Medicine and Pathology, Mayo Clinic
Rochester, Minnesota 55905, USA

Series Editor
L. H. Sobin
Head, WHO Collaborating Centre
for the International Histological Classification of Tumours
Armed Forces Institute of Pathology, Washington, DC, USA

First edition published by WHO in 1979 as No. 21 in the International Histological Classification of Tumours series

ISBN-13:978-3-540-56971-8 e-ISBN-13:978-3-642-84988-6
DOI: 10.1007/978-3-642-84988-6

Library of Congress Cataloging-in-Publication Data
Kleihues, P. (Paul) Histological typing of tumours of the central nervous system / P. Kleihues, P. C. Burger, and B. W. Scheithauer ; in collaboration with L. H. Sobin and pathologists in 14 countries. – 2nd ed. p. cm. – (International histological classification of tumours) Rev. ed. of: Histological typing of tumours of the central nervous system / K. J. Zülch, in collaboration with pathologists in 14 countries. 1979. Includes bibliographical references and index.
ISBN-13:978-3-540-56971-8

1. Central nervous system–Tumors–Histopathology–Atlases. 2. Tumors–Classification. I. Burger, Peter C., 1940– . II. Scheithauer, Bernd W., 1946– . III. Zülch, K. J. (Klaus Joachim), 1910– Histological typing of tumours of the central nervous system. IV. Title. V. Series: International histological classification of tumours (Unnumbered) [DNLM: 1. Neoplasms, Nervous Tissue–classification. 2. Neoplasms, Nervous Tissue–pathology. 3. Neoplasms, Nervous Tissue–pathology–atlases. 4. Central Nervous System Neoplasms–classification. 5. Central Nervous System Neoplasms–pathology. 6. Central Nervous System Neoplasms–pathology–atlases. QZ 15 K63h 1993] RC280.N43K54 1993 616.99'28'0012–dc20 DNLM/DLC for Library of Congress 93-25312 CIP

Reproduction of the figures: Gustav Dreher GmbH, Stuttgart

25/3145-5 4 3 2 1 0 – Printed on acid-free paper

Participants

Armstrong, D.L.D., Dr. [1]
Department of Pathology, Baylor College of Medicine, Houston, Texas 77030, USA

Barnard, R., Dr. [1]
Department of Pathology, Maida Vale Hospital, London W9 ITL, UK

Becker, L., Dr. [1,2]
Division of Neuropathology, The Hospital for Sick Children, University of Toronto, Toronto, Ontario MSG IX8, Canada

Bigner, D.D., Dr. [1]
Preuss Laboratory for Brain Tumor Research, Department of Pathology, Duke University Medical Center, Durham, North Carolina 27710, USA

Brucher, J.-M., Dr. [1,2]
Neuropathology Department, University of Louvain, 1200 Brussels, Belgium

Bruner, J.M., Dr. [1]
Department of Pathology, The University of Texas M. D. Anderson Cancer Center, Houston, Texas 77030, USA

Budka, H., Dr. [2]
Neurological Institute, University of Vienna, 1090 Vienna, Austria

Burger, P.C., Dr. [1,2]
Department of Pathology, Duke University Medical Center, Durham, North Carolina 27710, USA

Dastur, D.K., Dr. [2]
Department of Neuropathology & Applied Biology, Bombay Hospital, Bombay 400 020, India

Daumas-Duport, C., Dr. [1]
Department of Pathological Anatomy, Hôpital Sainte Anne, 75014 Paris, France

Davis, R.L., Dr. [1,2]
Department of Pathology, University of California School of Medicine, San Francisco, California 94143, USA

Earle, K.M., Dr. [1]
Our Lady of Lourdes Hospital, Lafayette, Louisiana 70501, USA

Fields, W.S., Dr. [1,2]
Department of Neuro-Oncology, The University of Texas M. D. Anderson Cancer Center, Houston, Texas 77030, USA

Giangaspero, F., Dr. [2]
Institute of Anatomy and Pathology, University of Bologna, 40138 Bologna, Italy

Gilles, F., Dr. [1]
Department of Pathology, Children's Hospital of Los Angeles, Los Angeles, California 90054, USA

Hassoun, J., Dr. [1,2]
Department of General Pathology and Neuropathology, Faculty of Medicine, 13385 Marseille Cedex 5, France

Ikuta, F., Dr. [2]
Brain Research Institute, Niigata University, Niigata City 951, Japan

Ishida, Y., Dr. [1,2]
Department of Pathology, Gunma University School of Medicine, Maebashi-shi, Gunma-Ken, Japan

Jänisch, W., Dr. [1,2]
Institute of Pathology, Humboldt University, 1000 Berlin, Germany

Jellinger, K., Dr. [1,2]
Ludwig Boltzmann Institute of Clinical Neurobiology, Lainz Hospital, 1130 Vienna, Austria

Kepes, J.J., Dr. [1,2]
Department of Pathology, University of Kansas Medical Center, Kansas City, Kansas 66103, USA

Kirkpatrick, J.B., Dr. [1]
Department of Pathology, The Methodist Hospital, Houston, Texas 77030, USA

Kleihues, P., Dr. [1,2]
Institute of Neuropathology, University Hospital, 8091 Zurich, Switzerland

Lantos, P.L., Dr. [2]
Department of Neuropathology, Institute of Psychiatry, London SE5 8AF, UK

Mennel, H.D., Dr. [2]
Department of Pathology, University of Marburg, 3550 Marburg/ Lahn, Germany

Mørk, S.J., Dr. [2]
The Gade Institute, Department of Pathology, Haukeland Hospital, University of Bergen, 5016 Bergen, Norway

Nelson, J.S., Dr. [2]
Department of Neuropathology, Armed Forces Institute of Pathology, Washington, DC 20306, USA

Rorke, L., Dr. [1,2]
The Children's Hospital of Philadelphia, Philadelphia, Pennsylvania 19104, USA

Rubinstein, L.J., Dr. [1]
Department of Pathology, Division of Neuropathology, University of Virginia School of Medicine, Charlottesville, Virginia 22908, USA

Scheithauer, B.W., Dr. [1,2]
Department of Laboratory Medicine and Pathology, Mayo Clinic, Rochester, Minnesota 55905, USA

Schiffer, D., Dr. [2]
Second Department of Neurology, University of Turin, 10126 Turin, Italy

Sobin, L.H., Dr. [1]
WHO Collaborating Center for International Histological Classification of Tumors, Armed Forces Institute of Pathology, Washington, DC 20306, USA

Szymas, J., Dr. [1]
Department of Clinical Pathomorphology, Academy of Medicine, 60 355 Poznan, Poland

Taratuto, A.L., Dr. [2]
Department of Neuropathology, Foundation of the Institute for Neurological Disorders in Children (FLENI), 1112 Buenos Aires, Argentina

VandenBerg, S.R., Dr. [2]
Division of Neuropathology, Department of Pathology, University of Virginia School of Medicine, Charlottesville, Virginia 22908, USA

Wechsler, W., Dr. [1,2]
Department of Neuropathology, Heinrich-Heine University, Dusseldorf, 4000 Dusseldorf, Germany

Weller, R.O., Dr. [2]
Laboratory of Neuropathology, University of Southampton, Southampton General Hospital, Southampton S09 4XY, UK

Yung, W.K.A., Dr. [1]
Department of Neuro-Oncology, The University of Texas M. D. Anderson Cancer Center, Houston, Texas 77030, USA

Zülch, K.-J., Dr. [1]
Max-Planck Institute for Brain Research, 5000 Cologne, Germany

---

1 Participant in the first meeting on brain tumour classification in Houston, Texas, USA, March 1988

2 Participant in the second meeting on brain tumour classification in Zurich, Switzerland, March 1990

General Preface to the Series

Among the prerequisites for comparative studies of cancer are international agreement on histological criteria for the definition and classification of cancer types and a standardized nomenclature. An internationally agreed classification of tumours, acceptable alike to physicians, surgeons, radiologists, pathologists and statisticians, would enable cancer workers in all parts of the world to compare their findings and would facilitate collaboration among them.

In a report published in 1952,[1] a subcommittee of the World Health Organization (WHO) Expert Committee on Health Statistics discussed the general principles that should govern the statistical classification of tumours and agreed that, to ensure the necessary flexibility and ease of coding, three separate classifications were needed according to (1) anatomical site, (2) histological type, and (3) degree of malignancy. A classification according to anatomical site is available in the International Classification of Diseases.[2]

In 1956, the WHO Executive Board passed a resolution[3] requesting the Director-General to explore the possibility that WHO might organize centres in various parts of the world and arrange for the collection of human tissues and their histological classification. The main purpose of such centres would be to

---

1 WHO (1952) WHO Technical Report Series. No. 53, 1952, p. 45

2 WHO (1977) Manual of the international statistical classification of diseases, injuries, and causes of death. 1975 version Geneva

3 WHO (1956) WHO Official Records. No. 68, p. 14 (resolution EB 17.R40)

4 WHO (1957) WHO Official Records. No. 79, p. 467 (resolution WHA 10.18)

develop histological definitions of cancer types and to facilitate the wide adoption of a uniform nomenclature. The resolution was endorsed by the Tenth World Health Assembly in May 1957.[4]

Since 1958, WHO has established a number of centres concerned with this subject. The result of this endeavor has been the International Histological Classification of Tumours, a multivolumed series whose first edition was published between 1967 and 1981. The present revised second edition aims to update the classification, reflecting progress in diagnosis and the relevance of tumour types to clinical and epidemiological features.

Preface to Histological Typing of Tumours of the Central Nervous System, Second Edition

The first edition of *Histological Typing of Tumours of the Central Nervous System*[1] was the result of a collaborative effort organized by WHO and conducted by the Collaborating Centre for Histological Classification of Tumours of the Central Nervous System established in 1970 at the Max-Planck Institute for Brain Research, Köln-Merheim, Federal Republic of Germany. This effort was coordinated by the late Professor Klaus Joachim Zülch. The classification was published under WHO auspices in 1979.

In order to keep the classification up to date, meetings were convened in 1988 at Houston, Texas, USA, and in 1990 at Zurich, Switzerland, to discuss proposals for revision (participants listed on pp. V–VII). The former meeting was organized by Professor William S. Fields and its deliberations were published in 1989[2]. At the latter meeting the present classification, definitions and explanatory notes were formulated and recommended for publication.

The histological classification of central nervous system tumours, which appears on pp. 3–8, contains the morphology

---

1 Zülch KJ (1979) Histological typing of tumours of the central nervous system, Geneva, World Health Organization (International Histological Classification of Tumours, No. 21)

2 Fields WS (ed) (1989) Primary brain tumors. A review of histologic classification. Springer, Berlin Heidelberg New York

3 World Health Organization (1990) International classification of diseases for oncology. Geneva

4 College of American Pathologists (1982) Systematized nomenclature of medicine. Chicago

code numbers of the International Classification of Diseases for Oncology (ICD-O)[3] and the Systematized Nomenclature of Medicine (SNOMED).[4]

It will, of course, be appreciated that this classification reflects the present state of knowledge, and modifications are likely to be needed as experience and new knowledge accumulate. Although the present classification has been adopted by the members, it necessarily represents a view from which some pathologists may wish to dissent. It is nevertheless hoped that, in the interests of international cooperation, all pathologists will try to use the classification as presented. Criticisms and suggestions for its improvement will be welcomed; these should be sent to the World Health Organization, Geneva, Switzerland.

The publications in the series International Histological Classification of Tumours are not intended to serve as textbooks but rather to promote the adoption of a uniform terminology that will facilitate and improve communication among cancer workers. For this reason the literature references have intentionally been kept to a minimum and readers should refer to standard works for more complete bibliographies.

Acknowledgements

The authors would like to thank Kathleen Laman and Dr. Figen Söylemezoglu for their help in preparing the photomicrographs and editing this volume.

Contents

Introduction

Although more than 12 years have passed since publication of the first WHO histological classification of central nervous system (CNS) tumours, the changes in this revised edition are not radical. Only one formerly recognized entity has been deleted: the monstrocellular sarcoma, because there is immunocytochemical evidence of its astrocytic nature. Several new tumour types have been added: the pleomorphic xanthoastrocytoma has been generally acknowledged for almost a decade; the neurocytoma has gradually evolved as a clinical–pathological entity; and two new entries, the dysembryoplastic neuroepithelial tumour and the desmoplastic infantile ganglioglioma, have only been characterized morphologically during the past few years.

We regard the classification as an international standard to facilitate communication and have tried to avoid current conceptual controversies. The majority of participants supported inclusion of the term "primitive neuroectodermal tumour" (PNET). However, because of our limited knowledge of the biology of embryonal CNS tumours, preference was given to use PNET selectively, rather than applying it to all small cell embryonal childhood tumours, irrespective of their histological phenotype.

Ependymomas and meningiomas now have new histological subtypes. Most of these are not associated with biological behaviour different from the parent tumour type, but their description will aid the practising pathologist to identify and classify these lesions.

Histological Typing

Following the philosophy of this WHO series, classification is based primarily on histological assessment of cell types and tissue patterns recognized by conventional light microscopy. However, we cannot neglect the advances brought to surgical pathology by immunocytochemistry. Therefore, relevant information on the expression of marker antigens is included where appropriate, e.g., glial fibrillary acidic protein (GFAP).

Histogenesis

Whenever convincing data point to the histogenesis of a tumour, this is used to define its placement within the classification scheme. Accordingly, the glioblastoma has been taken out of the group of "poorly differentiated and embryonal tumours", because there is increasing evidence that this lesion is of astrocytic nature and often presents the biological end point in the loss of differentiation typically associated with tumour progression in astrocytic neoplasms.

Despite the progress in immunocytochemistry, the histogenesis of some tumours has remained enigmatic. This is true for the astroblastoma and the polar spongioblastoma. Some participants regard these lesions merely as architectural patterns which may occur in a variety of gliomas, whereas others consider them as true clinical-pathological entities. To avoid any dogmatic decision, the working group recommended putting these lesions provisionally into a separate glioma group termed "neuroepithelial tumours of uncertain origin."

Grading

In the first edition of the WHO classification, the biological behaviour of CNS tumours was, in addition to describing histological evidence of differentiation or anaplasia, characterized by assigning a histological grade ranging from I (benign) to IV (malignant). This system was even applied to lesions typically occurring in only one or two form(s) of biological behaviour. Thus, the WHO grading, as it became known, was a malignancy scale ranging across a wide variety of intracranial neoplasms rather than a histological grading system. Nevertheless, it is now widely used, particularly in European countries. The participants, therefore, hold the view that this grading system should be continued on an optional basis. It is not an indispensible element of CNS tumour typing. Those who use it are advised to add the term "WHO" in order to avoid any confusion with other grading systems.

Histological Classification of Tumours of the Central Nervous System

1 Tumours of Neuroepithelial Tissue

1.1	***Astrocytic tumours***	
1.1.1	Astrocytoma	9400/3[a]
1.1.1.1	Variants: Fibrillary	9420/3
1.1.1.2	Protoplasmic	9410/3
1.1.1.3	Gemistocytic	9411/3
1.1.2	Anaplastic (malignant) astrocytoma	9401/3
1.1.3	Glioblastoma	9440/3
1.1.3.1	Variants: Giant cell glioblastoma	9441/3
1.1.3.2	Gliosarcoma	9442/3
1.1.4	Pilocytic astrocytoma	9421/3
1.1.5	Pleomorphic xanthoastrocytoma	9424/3
1.1.6	Subependymal giant cell astrocytoma (Tuberous sclerosis)	9384/1

1.2	***Oligodendroglial tumours***	
1.2.1	Oligodendroglioma	9450/3
1.2.2	Anaplastic (malignant) oligodendroglioma	9451/3

1.3	***Ependymal tumours***	
1.3.1	Ependymoma	9391/3
1.3.1.1	Variants: Cellular	
1.3.1.2	Papillary	9393/1
1.3.1.3	Clear cell	

[a] Morphology code of the International Classification of Diseases for Oncology (ICD-O) and Systematized Nomenclature of Medicine (SNOMED)

1.3.2	Anaplastic (malignant) ependymoma	9392/3
1.3.3	Myxopapillary ependymoma	9394/1
1.3.4	Subependymoma	9383/1
1.4	***Mixed gliomas***	
1.4.1	Oligo-astrocytoma	9382/3
1.4.2	Anaplastic (malignant) oligo-astrocytoma	
1.4.3	Others	
1.5	***Choroid plexus tumours***	
1.5.1	Choroid plexus papilloma	9390/0
1.5.2	Choroid plexus carcinoma	9390/3
1.6	***Neuroepithelial tumours of uncertain origin***	
1.6.1	Astroblastoma	9430/3
1.6.2	Polar spongioblastoma	9443/3
1.6.3	Gliomatosis cerebri	9381/3
1.7	***Neuronal and mixed neuronal-glial tumours***	
1.7.1	Gangliocytoma	9490/0
1.7.2	Dysplastic gangliocytoma of cerebellum (Lhermitte-Duclos)	9490/0
1.7.3	Desmoplastic infantile ganglioglioma	9505/0
1.7.4	Dysembryoplastic neuroepithelial tumour	
1.7.5	Ganglioglioma	9505/1
1.7.6	Anaplastic (malignant) ganglioglioma	9505/3
1.7.7	Central neurocytoma	9506/0
1.7.8	Paraganglioma of the filum terminale	8690/0
1.7.9	Olfactory neuroblastoma (Aesthesioneuroblastoma)	9522/3
1.7.9.1	Variant: Olfactory neuroepithelioma	9523/3
1.8	***Pineal parenchymal tumours***	
1.8.1	Pineocytoma	9361/1
1.8.2	Pineoblastoma	9362/3
1.8.3	Mixed / transitional pineal tumours	
1.9	***Embryonal tumours***	
1.9.1	Medulloepithelioma	9501/3

1.9.2	Neuroblastoma	9500/3
1.9.2.1	Variant: Ganglioneuroblastoma	9490/1
1.9.3	Ependymoblastoma	9392/3
1.9.4	Primitive neuroectodermal tumours (PNETs)	9473/3
1.9.4.1	Medulloblastoma	9470/3
1.9.4.1.1	Variants: Desmoplastic medulloblastoma	9471/3
1.9.4.1.2	Medullomyoblastoma	9472/3
1.9.4.1.3	Melanotic medulloblastoma	

2 Tumours of Cranial and Spinal Nerves

2.1	*Schwannoma (Neurilemmoma, Neurinoma)*	9560/0
2.1.1	Variants: Cellular	
2.1.2	Plexiform	
2.1.3	Melanotic	

2.2	*Neurofibroma*	9540/0
2.2.1	Circumscribed (solitary)	9540/0
2.2.2	Plexiform	9550/0

2.3	*Malignant peripheral nerve sheath tumour (MPNST)(Neurogenic sarcoma, Anaplastic neurofibroma, "Malignant schwannoma")*	9540/3
2.3.1	Variants: Epithelioid	
2.3.2	MPNST with divergent mesenchymal and/or epithelial differentiation	
2.3.3	Melanotic	

3 Tumours of the Meninges

3.1	*Tumours of meningothelial cells*	
3.1.1	Meningioma	9530/0
3.1.1.1	Variants: Meningothelial	9531/0
3.1.1.2	Fibrous (fibroblastic)	9532/0
3.1.1.3	Transitional (mixed)	9537/0

3.1.1.4	Psammomatous	9533/0
3.1.1.5	Angiomatous	9534/0
3.1.1.6	Microcystic	
3.1.1.7	Secretory	
3.1.1.8	Clear cell	
3.1.1.9	Chordoid	
3.1.1.10	Lymphoplasmacyte-rich	
3.1.1.11	Metaplastic	
3.1.2	Atypical meningioma	9530/1
3.1.3	Papillary meningioma	9538/1
3.1.4	Anaplastic (malignant) meningioma	9530/3

3.2	***Mesenchymal, non-meningothelial tumours***	
	Benign neoplasms	
3.2.1	Osteocartilaginous tumours	
3.2.2	Lipoma	8850/0
3.2.3	Fibrous histiocytoma	8830/0
3.2.4	Others	
	Malignant neoplasms	
3.2.5	Hemangiopericytoma	9150/3
3.2.6	Chondrosarcoma	9220/3
3.2.6.1	Variant: Mesenchymal chondrosarcoma	9240/3
3.2.7	Malignant fibrous histiocytoma	8830/3
3.2.8	Rhabdomyosarcoma	8900/3
3.2.9	Meningeal sarcomatosis	9539/3
3.2.10	Others	

3.3.	***Primary melanocytic lesions***	
3.3.1	Diffuse melanosis	57210
3.3.2	Melanocytoma	8726/1
3.3.3	Malignant melanoma	8720/3
3.3.3.1	Variant: Meningeal melanomatosis	8720/3

3.4	***Tumours of uncertain histogenesis***	
3.4.1	Haemangioblastoma (Capillary haemangioblastoma)	9161/1

4 Lymphomas and Haemopoietic Neoplasms

4.1	Malignant lymphomas	9590/3
4.2	Plasmacytoma	9731/3
4.3	Granulocytic sarcoma	9930/3
4.4	Others	

5 Germ Cell Tumours

5.1	Germinoma	9064/3
5.2	Embryonal carcinoma	9070/3
5.3	Yolk sac tumour (Endodermal sinus tumour)	9071/3
5.4	Choriocarcinoma	9100/3
5.5	Teratoma	9080/1
5.5.1	Immature	9080/3
5.5.2	Mature	9080/1
5.5.3	Teratoma with malignant transformation	9084/3
5.6	Mixed germ cell tumours	9085/3

6 Cysts and Tumour-like Lesions

6.1	Rathke cleft cyst	26500
6.2	Epidermoid cyst	33410
6.3	Dermoid cyst	9084/0
6.4	Colloid cyst of the third ventricle	33790
6.5	Enterogenous cyst	26660
6.6	Neuroglial cyst	26630
6.7	Granular cell tumour (Choristoma, Pituicytoma)	9580/0
6.8	Hypothalamic neuronal hamartoma	75500
6.9	Nasal glial heterotopia	26160
6.10	Plasma cell granuloma	43060

7 Tumours of the Sellar Region

7.1	Pituitary adenoma	8140/0
7.2	Pituitary carcinoma	8140/3

7.3	Craniopharyngioma	9350/1
7.3.1	Variants: Adamantinomatous	
7.3.2	Papillary	

8 Local Extensions from Regional Tumours

8.1	Paraganglioma (Chemodectoma)	8680/1
8.2	Chordoma	9370/0
8.3	Chondroma	9220/0
	Chondrosarcoma	9220/3
8.4	Carcinoma	8200/3

9 Metastatic Tumours 8000/6

10 Unclassified Tumours

Definitions and Explanatory Notes

1 Tumours of Neuroepithelial Tissue

Classification of the glial subset of neuroepithelial tumours is based on the predominant cell type. Admixture of other neoplastic cells occurs quite frequently and should not, unless substantial, lead to an excessive diagnosis of mixed gliomas.

Anaplasia is used as an operational term summarizing histopathological features typically associated with malignant biological behaviour and may include nuclear atypia, increased mitotic activity, atypical mitoses, cellular pleomorphism, vascular proliferation, and necrosis. Admittedly, the significance of some of these features may vary considerably in different tumour types. For example, nuclear atypia and extensive vascular proliferations indicate anaplasia and poor clinical prognosis in diffuse astrocytomas of the cerebral hemispheres but bear no such implications in a pilocytic astrocytoma. The same is true for ependymomas in which atypia, modest mitotic activity and even necrosis may lack prognostic significance.

1.1 Astrocytic Tumours

Tumours composed predominantly of neoplastic astrocytes.

Gliomas of astrocytic origin comprise neoplasms which vary widely in morphology and biological behaviour. Tumours listed below under Sects. 1.1.1–1.1.3 diffusely infiltrate surrounding brain structures whereas those listed under Sects. 1.1.4–1.1.6 are more circumscribed and show a lesser tendency towards tumour progression and increasing anaplasia.

1.1.1 Astrocytoma

A generic term applied to diffusely infiltrating tumours composed of well differentiated neoplastic astrocytes.

Microscopically, astrocytomas are ill-defined and show a consistent tendency to diffuse infiltration of the surrounding brain. Pre-existing cell types, e.g. neurons, are often entrapped. Phenotypically, neoplastic astrocytes may vary considerably with respect to size, prominence and disposition of cell processes, and the abundance of cytoplasmic glial filaments. The variants described below indicate the predominant cell type; admixture of other types of neoplastic astrocytes is common.

Macroscopically, astrocytomas are ill-defined and appear yellow–white and homogeneous. Single or multiple cysts containing a clear fluid may be seen. Diffuse infiltration with gradual incorporation of pre-existing cells often leads to an enlargement and distortion, but not destruction, of the invaded anatomical structures, e.g. cortex and compact myelinated pathways. Mitotic activity is absent.

Astrocytomas typically occur in early adult life, with a peak incidence in the fourth and fifth decades. They may be located at any site in the central nervous system (CNS), including the spinal cord, but preferentially involve the cerebral hemispheres. In children, they often occur in the pons.

Biological behaviour: Well-differentiated astrocytomas grow slowly and correspond histologically to Grade II. However, due to incomplete surgical resection, they almost always recur. Also, there is an inherent tendency for progression to anaplastic astrocytoma and, eventually, to glioblastoma. This is particularly true for the gemistocytic variant which is associated with a poor prognosis.

1.1.1.1 Fibrillary Astrocytoma (Figs. 1, 2)

This is by far the most frequent variant of astrocytoma. Cell density is low to moderate. Astrocytic nuclei are hyperchromatic, oval to irregular, without mitotic activity. On sections stained with haematoxylin-eosin (H&E), the cytoplasm is often scant and barely discernible. This is a typical feature in biopsies in which isolated tumour cells lie within intact parenchyma. In more cellular lesions, numerous cell processes form a loose fibrillary matrix, occasionally with microcyst formation. Glial fibrillary acidic protein (GFAP) is consistently expressed in such areas.

1.1.1.2 Protoplasmic Astrocytoma (Fig. 3)

This rare variant is characterized by neoplastic astrocytes showing a small cell body with few, flaccid processes with a low content of glial filaments. Accordingly, GFAP immunostaining is scant. Microcyst formation is common. This variant appears to be often superficial in location and cystic.

1.1.1.3 Gemistocytic Astrocytoma (Fig. 4)

A variant of astrocytoma predominantly composed of gemistocytic astrocytes. Tumour cells show large eosinophilic cell bodies, angular shape and short, stout, randomly oriented, GFAP-positive processes forming a coarse fibrillary network. Nuclei are round to oval and usually eccentric. Perivascular lymphocyte cuffing is more frequent in this than in other astrocytomas.

1.1.2 Anaplastic (Malignant) Astrocytoma (Fig. 5)

An astrocytoma with focal or diffuse anaplasia, e.g. increased cellularity, pleomorphism, nuclear atypia and mitotic activity.

Vascular proliferation and necrosis are absent. GFAP immunostaining may vary but usually resembles that of low grade astrocytomas.

Biological behaviour: Anaplastic astrocytomas correspond histologically to Grade III. Such tumours show an inherent and often rapid tendency to progress, ultimately with transition to glioblastoma.

1.1.3 Glioblastoma (Figs. 6–9)

An anaplastic, often cellular brain tumour composed of poorly differentiated, fusiform, round or pleomorphic cells and occasional multinucleated giant cells. Essential for the histological diagnosis is the presence of prominent vascular proliferation and/or necrosis.

Mitotic activity and the occurrence of atypical mitoses vary considerably. Pseudopalisading around areas of tumour necrosis is often present. Expression of GFAP varies considerably and may be absent focally. Many glioblastomas contain areas with differentiated neoplastic astrocytes, indicating their astrocytic nature and frequent evolution from low grade or anaplastic astrocytoma. Macroscopically, they may appear deceptively circumscribed, typically with a tendency to varied coloration due to degeneration, necrosis and occasional haemorrhage.

This common, highly anaplastic brain tumour occurs in late adult life, with a peak incidence between 45 and 60 years. It is typically located in the cerebral hemispheres. Although most are frontotemporal in location, glioblastomas occasionally manifest at other sites, e.g. cerebellum, brain stem and spinal cord.

Biological behaviour: Glioblastomas correspond histologically to Grade IV.

1.1.3.1 Giant Cell Glioblastoma (Fig. 10)

A glioblastoma with a marked predominance of bizarre, multinucleated giant cells and, on occasion, an abundant stromal reticulin network. GFAP expression may be highly variable. Giant cell glioblastomas tend to be macroscopically well-circumscribed.

1.1.3.2 Gliosarcoma (Figs. 11, 12)

A glioblastoma admixed with a sarcomatous component. The latter is presumed to originate from malignant transformation of the hyperplastic vascular elements typically observed in glioblastomas. The sarcomatous tissue often resembles fibrosarcoma, but pleomorphism can be considerable. The sarcoma may predominate in some cases. Reticulin stains and immunoreactivity for GFAP or S-100 protein readily distinguish the components.

1.1.4 Pilocytic Astrocytoma (Figs. 13–16)

A circumscribed astrocytoma composed, at least in part, of bipolar, fusiform or 'piloid' cells with dense fibrillation. Tumour cells tend to form compact parallel bundles. Particularly common is a biphasic pattern in which pilocytic areas are intimately associated with a loosely structured microcystic component consisting of protoplasmic, poorly fibrillated neoplastic astrocytes.

Hyperchromatic, bizarre nuclei may be present and are not, in the absence of significant mitotic activity, associated with a poor prognosis. GFAP expression is always demonstrable, although to a varying degree. The microcysts apparently coalesce to larger cysts which may, when situated in the posterior fossa, displace the vermis or large parts of the cerebellar hemisphere. The stroma consists of irregularly disposed blood vessels which may be hyalinized. Glomeruloid capillary or even endothelial proliferation is not uncommon, both within the tumour and in the wall of cysts, but does not signify malignancy. Elongated eosinophilic, club-shaped structures (Rosenthal fibres) and eosinophilic intracytoplasmic protein droplets ("granular bodies") are histopathological hallmarks of this neoplasm. Calcification may also be seen but is usually inconspicuous. Local invasion of the subarachnoid space is frequent and may be accompanied by a desmoplastic leptomeningeal reaction, but does not indicate malignancy.

In contrast to the above mentioned diffuse astrocytic tumours, the pilocytic astrocytoma is more circumscribed, expands into the surrounding brain only slowly, and very rarely shows a tendency for progression to anaplasia. This tumour occurs mainly in children, with a peak incidence around the age 10 years, and in young adults. Pilocytic astrocytomas are typically located in midline structures, e.g. optic nerve (optic nerve glioma), third ventricle, thalamus, median temporal lobe, brain stem and in the cerebellum ('cystic and solid cerebellar astrocytoma'). The cerebral hemispheres are affected less frequently.

Biological behaviour: This slowly growing tumour corresponds histologically to Grade I. Malignant transformation occurs very rarely, in which case the tumour is categorized as an anaplastic (pilocytic) astrocytoma (Grade III).

1.1.5 **Pleomorphic Xanthoastrocytoma** (Figs. 17–19)

An astrocytoma with a mixture of pleomorphic tumour cells, ranging from ordinary fibrillary astrocytes to giant, multinucleated forms. The latter typically contain lipid vacuoles; thus they are xanthomatous, but express GFAP.

The superficial, in particular the leptomeningeal, portions of these tumours, exhibit a dense intercellular reticulin network due to the presence of pericellular basement membranes. Mitoses are rare and necrosis as well as vascular proliferation are absent. This rare variant of astrocytoma often occurs in children or young adults and affects the cerebral hemispheres, particularly the temporal lobe. It is typically superficial in location, shows an intimate relation to the meninges and may be associated with an underlying cyst.

Biological behaviour: Despite its pleomorphic appearance, this neoplasm is usually rather well-demarcated. A generally favourable prognosis justifies its inclusion in Grade II gliomas. A minority of pleomorphic xanthoastrocytomas do, however, progress to anaplastic astrocytoma (Grade III) or glioblastoma (Grade IV).

1.1.6 **Subependymal Giant Cell Astrocytoma (Tuberous Sclerosis)** (Figs. 20, 21)

A circumscribed, usually calcified intraventricular tumour arising from the walls of the lateral ventricles. It is composed mainly of large plump cells resembling astrocytes.

Perivascular pseudopalisading and clustering of tumour cells are common features. The vesicular, often eccentric nuclei may contain prominent nucleoli. GFAP expression is variable but usually demonstrable. Tumour cells occasionally express neuronal marker antigens. Mitoses are rare or absent. These lesions often overlie the head of the caudate nucleus, may occlude the foramen of Monro, and typically occur in young patients as part of the tuberous sclerosis complex.

Biological behaviour: The tumour grows very slowly, is often static, and may be cured by surgical resection. It corresponds histologically to Grade I.

1.2 Oligodendroglial Tumours

1.2.1 Oligodendroglioma (Figs. 22–24)

A tumour composed predominantly of neoplastic oligodendrocytes.

Microscopically, most oligodendrogliomas are moderately cellular. Tumour cells typically exhibit spherical, often hyperchromatic nuclei surrounded by artefactually swollen, clear cytoplasm. A well-defined plasma membrane lends a so-called honeycomb or fried egg appearance. Mitoses are infrequent. The stroma mainly consists of delicate, capillary-sized blood vessels, often arranged in an acutely branching or 'chicken wire' pattern. Endothelial hyperplasia is absent or mild. Focal calcifications are a histopathological hallmark of oligodendrogliomas and are often most conspicuous in the peripheral zone of infiltration. Immunoreactivity to S-100 protein and Leu 7 is typically encountered, but to date, no specific immunocytochemical marker is available for oligodendrogliomas. It should be noted that in up to 50% of tumours, a fraction of otherwise typical neoplastic oligodendrocytes express GFAP.

This slowly growing neoplasm usually occurs in adults and preferentially affects the cerebral white matter and basal ganglia. Cortical extension is frequent. Primary lesions may be macroscopically defined and greyish-pink, with a tendency to invasion of the leptomeninges.

Biological behaviour: Oligodendrogliomas usually develop slowly over a period of years during which many are associated with seizures as the only clinical manifestation. Postoperative survival varies considerably, but tumour progression to frank anaplasia occurs less frequently than in astrocytomas. Histologically, oligodendrogliomas correspond to Grade II.

1.2.2 Anaplastic (Malignant) Oligodendroglioma (Fig. 25)

An oligodendroglioma with focal or diffuse anaplasia, e.g. high cellularity, nuclear polymorphism and brisk mitotic activity. Occasional multinucleated giant cells, vascular proliferation, mitotic activity and foci of necrosis may also be seen. Anaplastic oligodendrogliomas often contain a significant admixture of neoplastic astrocytes.

Biological behaviour: These neoplasms correspond histologically to Grade III but may progress to a highly anaplastic tumour that may be morphologically indistinguishable from glioblastoma (Grade IV).

1.3 Ependymal Tumours

1.3.1 Ependymoma (Figs. 26, 27)

A tumour composed predominantly of neoplastic ependymal cells.

Microscopically, ependymomas are moderately cellular and exhibit low mitotic activity. Histological hallmarks include perivascular pseudorosettes and ependymal rosettes, the latter being less frequent but more diagnostic. GFAP expression varies considerably and, if present, is usually restricted to the radiating cell processes of perivascular pseudorosettes. Occasional mitoses, nuclear atypia and even foci of necrosis may be seen, but are not necessarily indicative of malignancy.

Ependymomas are thought to develop from the ependymal or subependymal cells surrounding the ventricles and the central canal of the spinal cord as well as from ependymal clusters in the filum terminale. Intracranial ependymomas occur predominantly in children and tend to fill the ventricular lumen. Ependymomas of the fourth ventricle may extend through the foramina of Luschka and Magendi to gain access to the subarachnoid space and basal cisterns. Although ependymomas are usually solid and demarcated, only limited infiltration of adjacent brain structures is observed. Spinal ependymomas are usually diagnosed in adults and are preferentially located in the lumbosacral region.

Biological behaviour: Slowly growing and usually well-delineated from adjacent brain structures, ependymomas correspond histologically to Grade II.

1.3.1.1 Cellular Ependymoma

A variant of ependymoma with conspicuous cellularity but often less prominent pseudorosette or rosette formation.

1.3.1.2 Papillary Ependymoma (Fig. 28)

A rare variant of ependymoma which may mimic the histological pattern of choroid plexus papilloma. Distinguishing features are GFAP-positive cell processes radiating toward central vessels, a pseudostratified arrangement of tumour cells, the presence of a glial matrix and the absence of a prominent basement membrane separating cells from the underlying vascular stroma.

1.3.1.3 Clear Cell Ependymoma (Fig. 29)

An ependymoma dominated by tumour cells exhibiting swollen, clear cytoplasm and well-defined plasma membranes. This rare variant may be confused with oligodendroglioma, neurocytoma or metastatic renal cell carcinoma.

1.3.2 Anaplastic (Malignant) Ependymoma (Fig. 30)

An ependymal tumour with histological evidence of anaplasia, e.g. high cellularity, variable nuclear atypia, marked mitotic activity and often prominent vascular proliferation.

Necrosis may be widespread but is of less diagnostic significance. Tumour progression may be paralleled by the loss of typical architectural features, e.g. perivascular pseudorosettes and true rosettes, but evolution to a glioblastoma phenotype is rare. Seeding via cerebrospinal fluid (CSF) pathways may occur.

Biological behaviour: Anaplastic ependymomas correspond histologically to Grade III.

1.3.3 Myxopapillary Ependymoma (Figs. 31, 32)

A variant of ependymoma that occurs almost exclusively in the region of the cauda equina and originates from the filum terminale. It is histologically characterized by cuboidal to elongated tumour cells arranged in a perivascular papillary pattern around central cores of mucinous or hyalinized perivascular stroma.

Tumour cells may also surround pools of mucin but their glial nature can usually be confirmed by immunoreactivity for GFAP. Secondary involvement of the conus medullaris is common.

Biological behaviour: Although complete surgical resection can only be achieved in those instances wherein the tumour forms an intact, sausage-shaped expansion of the filum, this slowly growing neoplasm is biologically a benign form of ependymoma and corresponds histologically to Grade I.

1.3.4 Subependymoma (Figs. 33, 34)

A nodular tumour composed of nests of ependymal cells in a dense glial fibrillary matrix.

Microscopically, subependymomas consist of clusters of ependymal cells with round nuclei, surrounded by broad swirls of glial processes. A variable admixture of fibrillary astrocytes is often seen. Mitoses are absent or rare. Microcysts and calcifications are common features. Vascular hyalinization and foci of haemosiderin deposition are common in larger tumours and indicate previous haemorrhage. Occasional lesions display histopathological features of both subependymoma and ependymoma.

The majority of subependymomas present as well-delineated, firm, occasionally multiple nodules in the fourth and lateral ventricles of adult patients. Most are asymptomatic.

Biological behaviour: Despite their usually slow growth, a fraction of subependymomas causes symptoms by obstructing CSF pathways. Histologically, subependymomas correspond to Grade I. Mixed subependymoma – ependymomas may behave more like ependymomas (Grade II).

1.4 Mixed Gliomas

During the past decade, it has been increasingly recognized that, in addition to monotypic gliomas, there are neoplasms which exhibit a blend of two or more neoplastic glial cell types.

1.4.1 Oligo-astrocytoma (Fig. 35)

A tumour with a conspicuous mixture of neoplastic oligodendrocytes and astrocytes, either diffusely intermingled or separated into distinct areas.

Tumours containing cells with oligodendroglial nuclei and small eccentric GFAP-positive cell bodies are not considered to be mixed gliomas.

Biological behaviour: Histologically, mixed oligo-astrocytomas correspond to Grade II.

1.4.2 Anaplastic (Malignant) Oligo-astrocytoma

An oligo-astrocytoma with histological evidence of anaplasia, e.g. increased cellularity, nuclear atypia and brisk mitotic activity. Vascular proliferation and focal necrosis may be seen.

Histologically, anaplastic oligo-astrocytomas correspond to Grade III.

1.4.3 Others

This category allows for the inclusion of other, albeit rare, mixed gliomas containing additional cellular components, e.g. neoplastic ependymal cells.

1.5 Choroid Plexus Tumours

1.5.1 Choroid Plexus Papilloma (Fig. 36)

An epithelial tumour of the choroid plexus of the cerebral ventricles. It is composed of a simple or pseudostratified layer of cuboidal to columnar cells resting upon a basement membrane overlying papillary, vascularized connective tissue cores.

In small biopsies, it may be difficult to distinguish a papilloma from the more orderly normal choroid plexus or from papillary ependymoma (see Sect. 1.3.1.2). Cytological atypia, occasional mitoses and a rare focus of necrosis may be present. Demonstration of transthyretin immunoreactivity, though not specific, may aid in the differential diagnosis versus other neoplasms with papillary structures. An oncocytic variant is occasionally observed.

Biological behaviour: This benign, slowly growing neoplasm may cause obstruction of CSF pathways or may itself produce CSF in excess. Choroid plexus papillomas may seed into the CSF but metastatic growth at distant sites is unusual. Limited infiltration of underlying brain parenchyma may occur but does not appear to affect prognosis. Malignant transformation is rare. Histologically, choroid plexus papillomas correspond to Grade I.

1.5.2 Choroid Plexus Carcinoma (Fig. 37)

A choroid plexus tumour with histological evidence of anaplasia, e.g. increased mitotic activity, nuclear atypia, loss of papillary differentiation with transition to patternless cellular sheets and necrosis.

This rare variant may be difficult to distinguish from metastatic carcinoma to the choroid plexus. Immunoreactivity for cytokeratin, vimentin, S-100 protein, transthyretin and carboanhydrase C, but usually not for epithelial membrane antigen (EMA) typifies choroid tumours. Carcinoembryonic antigen (CEA) has proved to be unreliable in the distinction from metastatic carcinoma.

Biological behaviour: Seeding via CSF pathways may occur. Histologically, choroid plexus carcinomas correspond to Grade III.

1.6 Neuroepithelial Tumours of Uncertain Origin

This newly created category contains neuroepithelial neoplasms the histogenesis of which has not been established. Some members of the WHO working group maintain the view that these neoplasms are more likely to be ordinary gliomas exhibiting distinct histopathological and growth patterns, rather than true clinical pathological entities.

1.6.1 Astroblastoma (Fig. 38)

A glial neoplasm having a distinctive pattern of perivascular astrocytic cells with broad, non-tapering processes radiating towards a central blood vessel. These cells strongly express GFAP.

Astroblastic features may also be focally present in low (Grade II) and high grade (Grade III) astrocytomas and in glioblastomas.

1.6.2 Polar Spongioblastoma (Fig. 39)

A very rare childhood tumour, predominantly composed of unipolar or bipolar glial cells, the nuclei of which are arranged in parallel, thus forming a typical palisading pattern.

These neoplasms may, in other areas, exhibit the histopathological features of pilocytic astrocytoma or of oligodendroglioma. Their biological behaviour is variable. The polar spongioblastoma should not be confused with primitive neuroectodermal tumours, particularly cerebellar medulloblastomas, exhibiting palisading patterns.

1.6.3 Gliomatosis Cerebri

Diffuse neoplastic glial cell infiltration of the brain involving several cerebral lobes and, on occasion, infratentorial structures and the spinal cord.

Histopathologically, the tumour cells vary in shape from oval to elongated and with respect to atypia and mitotic activity. They appear to migrate widely along myelinated pathways without destruction of the invaded brain parenchyma. The frequent lack of immunoreactivity to GFAP may reflect loss of differentiation. Focal transformation to glioblastoma may occur. Macroscopically, gliomatosis cerebri is ill-defined and often only suggested by a diffuse enlargement of infiltrated CNS structures. Since the diagnosis of gliomatosis cerebri requires the involvement of several lobes, it requires neuroradiological correlation and usually cannot be made on the basis of a single surgical biopsy.

Biological behaviour: Gliomatosis cerebri corresponds histologically to Grade III or IV.

1.7 Neuronal and Mixed Neuronal–Glial Tumours

1.7.1 **Gangliocytoma** (Fig. 40)

A tumour composed predominantly of neoplastic though mature ganglion cells with a minor component of supportive, non-neoplastic glial cells.

Gangliocytomas are often of low cellularity and may be difficult to distinguish from neuronal heterotopias. Neoplastic ganglion cells are highly differentiated but can usually be distinguished from their normal counterparts by their dysplastic, occasionally bizarre appearance. The presence of binucleate or multinucleate neurons is regarded as diagnostic. Macroscopically, gangliocytomas are well-delineated, and are occasionally associated with calcification.

These slowly growing neoplasms usually occur in children and young adults. They may be located in any region of the CNS but the temporal lobe is their preferential site. When located in the hypothalamic region, they may cause endocrine hyperfunction.

Biological behaviour: Gangliocytomas grow slowly, do not undergo anaplastic change and correspond histologically to Grade I.

1.7.2 **Dysplastic Gangliocytoma of Cerebellum (Lhermitte–Duclos)** (Figs. 41, 42)

A very rare, tumour–like neuronal lesion of the cerebellum, with distinct dysplastic features. It consists of a diffuse cortical accumulation of abnormally large, dysplastic granular cells which superficially resemble Purkinje neurons.

Normal granular neurons are often reduced in number. Macroscopically, this lesion is ill-defined and mimics normal cerebellum although the folia are enlarged and occasionally distorted. An association with malformations, e.g. megalencephaly and leontiasis ossea, has been reported, as has familial occurrence.

Biological behaviour: This slowly growing lesion is benign, although late recurrences have been noted. Histologically, it corresponds to Grade I.

1.7.3 Desmoplastic Infantile Ganglioglioma (Figs. 43, 44)

A mixed neuronal–glial neoplasm of infancy with a distinct desmoplastic component. It is characterized by a dense fibrous stroma containing an admixture of neuroepithelial cells displaying astrocytic and neuronal differentiation.

Ganglion cells of the desmoplastic infantile ganglioglioma (DIG) may be small, plump, without Nissl substance and only identifiable by their immunoreactivity for neuronal markers, e.g. synaptophysin or neurofilament protein. The astrocytes are often elongated and express GFAP. Occasional mitoses may be seen. A focal admixture of small neuroepithelial cells of primitive appearance may also be present. Similar tumours with desmoplasia and neoplastic astrocytes have been described without a distinct neuronal component ('desmoplastic astrocytoma of infancy' or 'superficial dural astrocytoma'). The DIG usually occurs in children below the age of two years, is preferentially located superficially in the cerebral hemispheres, and appears macroscopically as a large, fibrous mass.

Biological behaviour: Although the DIG is usually large at diagnosis, it grows slowly and surgical resection is often followed by a favourable course. Histologically, it corresponds to Grade I.

1.7.4 Dysembryoplastic Neuroepithelial Tumour (Figs. 45, 46)

A benign, supratentorial mixed glial–neuronal neoplasm characterized by its intracortical location, multinodular architecture and heterogeneous cellular composition. Cortical dysplasia may also be present.

This tumour typically consists of neoplastic oligodendrocytes, neurons and, less prominently, of astrocytes. The dysembryoplastic neuroepithelial tumour (DNT) may be confused with a mixed oligoastrocytoma since the neuronal component may be rather inconspicuous. The cerebral cortex between nodules often shows an increase in oligodendroglial cells as well as of neurons which appear to float in spaces among them without associated satellitosis. Atypia is minimal and mitoses are rare or absent. Cystic change or calcification may occur. This recently recognized entity is usually diagnosed in children and young adults with a long history of partial complex seizures.

Biological behaviour: The DNT grows slowly, if at all, and does not recur after surgical resection. Histologically, it corresponds to Grade I.

1.7.5 Ganglioglioma (Figs. 47, 48)

A benign tumour composed of neoplastic astrocytes (rarely oligodendrocytes) and ganglion cells.

With respect to age distribution and location, this lesion resembles gangliocytomas (see Sect. 1.7.1). However, gangliogliomas are more often cystic and possess a truly neoplastic glial component. A striking mesenchymal component and perivascular lymphocytic infiltrates may be present.

Biological behaviour: It is generally agreed that the biology of these neoplasms is determined by the glial component. Histologically, gangliogliomas correspond to Grade I or Grade II.

1.7.6 Anaplastic (Malignant) Ganglioglioma

A rare variant of ganglioglioma in which the glial component shows distinct features of anaplasia, e.g. excessive atypia, increased mitotic activity, vascular proliferation and necrosis.

Biological behaviour: Anaplastic gangliogliomas correspond histologically to Grade III.

1.7.7 Central Neurocytoma (Figs. 49, 50)

An intraventricular tumour composed of uniform round cells with immunohistochemical and ultrastructural features of neuronal differentiation.

Histologically, neurocytomas are composed of uniform round cells, often with clear cytoplasm and easily recognizable cell membranes — a pattern mimicking neoplastic oligodendrocytes. Focally, perivascular, nuclei-free zones are reminiscent of ependymoma. An additional characteristic feature is the presence of finely fibrillar processes forming areas resembling neuropil. The neuronal differentiation of the central neurocytoma is evident from the electron microscopic identification of axons, synapses, microtubules and neurosecretory granules, as well as by their immunoreactivity for neuronal marker proteins, e.g. synaptophysin. Co-expression of GFAP has been observed.

This recently recognized entity usually occurs in young adults and is located in the lateral ventricles, typically in the region of the foramen of Monro and septum pellucidum. It grows primarily within the ventricular cavity and may obstruct CSF pathways.

Biological behaviour: Following surgical resection, this lesion carries a favourable prognosis. Histologically, central neurocytomas correspond to Grade I.

1.7.8 Paraganglioma of the Filum Terminale

A benign tumour, identical to extra-adrenal paraganglioma, but originating in the filum terminale or, rarely, from intradural lumbosacral nerve roots.

This slowly growing neoplasm usually occurs in adults and shows the typical histopathological pattern of paraganglioma, i.e. polygonal to elongated, delicately granulated cells, often abutting onto the vasculature. Vessels are abundant and the cells form an alveolar or *Zellballen* pattern. The diagnosis is confirmed by silver stains, immunoreactivity for chromogranin, somatostatin or synaptophysin or by electron microscopic identification of dense-core granules and processes with microtubules. Some lesions also contain ganglion cells ("gangliocytic paraganglioma").

Biological behaviour: Paragangliomas correspond histologically to Grade I.

1.7.9 Olfactory Neuroblastoma (Aesthesioneuroblastoma) (Fig. 51)

A tumour predominantly composed of immature neuronal cells presumed to be derived from precursor cells of the nasal neuroepithelium.

Histologically, the olfactory neuroblastoma is composed of nodules and irregular islands of neuroblasts which lie within a richly vascularized stroma. Neuroblastic (Homer Wright) rosettes are infrequent. Mitoses are present but vary in number. Immunohistochemistry reveals the expression of neuronal markers, e.g. neurofilament protein and synaptophysin. Electron microscopically, the neuronal nature is evident from the presence of numerous dense-core vesicles, neurites or microtubules. This tumour occurs preferentially in young adults and is typically located in the vault of the nose, often with infiltration of the cribriform plate.

Biological behaviour: Olfactory neuroblastomas tend to infiltrate adjacent structures, particularly the intracranial space via the cribriform plate. Invasion of accessory sinuses and orbit may be seen, as well as metastases to regional lymph nodes. Histologically, olfactory neuroblastomas correspond to Grade III.

1.7.9.1 Olfactory Neuroepithelioma (Aesthesioneuroepithelioma)

A rare variant of olfactory neuroblastoma characterized by neuronal and glandular differentiation. It shows immunoreactivity to both neuronal and epithelial marker proteins. This as well as olfactory neuroblastoma should be distinguished from neuro-endocrine carcinoma of the nose and paranasal sinuses.

1.8 Pineal Parenchymal Tumours

Pineal parenchymal tumours exhibit a continuous spectrum of differentiation, ranging from highly malignant pineoblastoma to the well-differentiated pineocytoma which carries a more favourable prognosis.

1.8.1 Pineocytoma (Fig. 52)

A rare, differentiated tumour composed of neoplastic pineal parenchymal cells.

Pineocytomas are moderately cellular with a delicate connective tissue stroma and a sheet-like to lobulated pattern. Pineocytic rosettes resembling enlarged Homer Wright rosettes are a common feature. Immunocytochemical analyses consistently reveal immunoreactivity to synaptophysin. Some lesions show progressive neuronal differentiation with the development of mature ganglion cells. Retinal differentiation may manifest by immunoreactivity for retinal S-antigen or, more rarely, fleurette formation. Occasional pineocytomas also show evidence of astrocytic differentiation. This lesion usually affects young adults.

Biological behaviour: Pineocytomas grow slowly and are well demarcated but may become symptomatic by compressing adjacent brain structures, including the aqueduct, with consequent hydrocephalus. Cerebrospinal spread via the CSF is very infrequent. Histologically, pineocytomas correspond to Grade II.

1.8.2 Pineoblastoma (Fig. 53)

A rare, malignant embryonal tumour assumed to originate from precursor cells of the pineal gland.

Pineoblastomas are highly cellular, with increased mitotic activity and a general histological appearance resembling that of cerebellar medulloblastomas, including the presence of neuroblastic Homer Wright rosettes. Immunohistochemcal evidence of neuronal or glial differentiation is less frequent than in pineocytomas.

This tumour typically occurs in children or young adults. It is ill-defined and usually causes symptoms by obstructing CSF pathways or by infiltrating adjacent brain structures.

Biological behaviour: Pineoblastomas are highly malignant and tend to metastasize via the CSF. They correspond histologically to Grade IV.

1.8.3 Mixed Pineocytoma/Pineoblastoma

A tumour containing areas composed of immature (pineoblastic) and differentiated (pineocytic) neoplastic cells. More often, these neoplasms exhibit cytological and histological features intermediate between these extremes.

1.9 Embryonal Tumours

During recent years studies of the histogenesis of embryonal CNS tumours have led to the new term "primitive neuroectodermal tumour" (PNET). The conceptual basis for this nomenclature is the assumption that PNETs share a common progenitor cell population which may undergo malignant transformation at various levels of the CNS, leading to tumours with similar morphology and biology. Some authors have proposed that all embryonal CNS tumours should be named PNETs, irrespective of their morphology and prevailing line of differentiation. Most members of the working group held the view that the WHO classification should avoid this controversy and voted to use the diagnosis PNET as a generic term for cerebellar medulloblastomas and for neoplasms which are morphologically indistinguishable from the medulloblastoma but are located at other sites in the CNS.

1.9.1 Medulloepithelioma (Fig. 54)

A very rare, malignant, embryonal tumour resembling primitive medullary epithelium of the neural tube.

Medulloepitheliomas consist of glandular structures lined by columnar to pseudostratified tumour cells, surrounded by a basement membrane. Tubular and papillary patterns may also be seen. In addition, they show a tendency to neuronal, glial or even specialized mesenchymal differentiation. Their malignant nature is reflected by high mitotic activity, necrosis and infiltrative growth.

Biological behaviour: This childhood neoplasm infiltrates adjacent brain structures and has a tendency to metastasize via the CSF. It corresponds histopathologically to Grade IV.

1.9.2 Neuroblastoma

A rare, malignant embryonal tumour composed of neuroblasts or cells with limited neuronal differentiation.

These highly cellular lesions contain cells with round to oval nuclei and a scant cytoplasm. Their neuronal character is reflected by the occurrence of neuroblastic (Homer Wright) rosettes and the consistent expression, by the vast majority of tumour cells, of neuronal proteins, e.g. neurofilament protein and synaptophysin. Ultrastructurally, tumour cells show processes containing microtubules as well as neurosecretory granules.

These childhood neoplasms are often well demarcated and deeply situated in the cerebral hemispheres but may be located at any site in the CNS, including the spinal cord and cauda equina.

Biological behaviour: Histologically, CNS neuroblastomas correspond to Grade IV.

1.9.2.1 Ganglioneuroblastoma (Fig. 55)

A neuroblastoma with focally advanced neuronal differentiation, including mature ganglion cells.

Assuming that the undifferentiated tumour cells determine the overall biological behaviour, ganglioneuroblastomas should, like neuroblastomas, be considered as Grade IV.

1.9.3 Ependymoblastoma (Fig. 56)

A rare, malignant embryonal tumour with distinct ependymal differentiation.

It is composed largely of undifferentiated cells, accompanied by numerous, surprisingly well-formed ependymoblastic rosettes. The latter are multilayered, true rosettes with a lumen. Ependymoblastomas are further characterized by high cellularity, marked mitotic activity and occasional areas of necrosis. This childhood tumour appears to be well-delineated macroscopically but histologically it invades the surrounding brain tissue and has a tendency for metastatic spread via the CSF.

Biological behaviour: Histologically, ependymoblastomas correspond to Grade IV.

1.9.4 Primitive Neuroectodermal Tumours (PNETs) (Fig. 57)

Small cell, malignant tumours of childhood with predominant location in the cerebellum and a noted capacity for divergent differentiation, including neuronal, astrocytic, ependymal, muscular and melanotic.

1.9.4.1 **Medulloblastoma** (Figs. 58–60)

A malignant, embryonal childhood tumour located in the cerebellum and composed of densely packed cells with round to oval, or carrot-shaped nuclei and scanty cytoplasm.

There is notable, though variable, mitotic activity and occasional areas of necrosis may be seen. Neuroblastic Homer Wright rosettes can be identified in up to 40% of cases. Immunocytochemical analyses have shown that the majority of medulloblastomas express neuronal marker proteins, including synaptophysin and neurofilament protein. Occasionally, maturation leads to the appearance of ganglion cells. Astrocytic differentiation is less common and usually restricted to focal GFAP expression. Ependymal features are very rare.

From their predominant site of origin, the vermis, medulloblastomas infiltrate adjacent brain structures including the cerebellar peduncles and, on occasion, the brain stem. They show a consistent tendency to invade the meninges and to spread via CSF pathways.

Biological behaviour: Despite considerable therapeutic progress in the treatment of medulloblastomas and related PNETs, these lesions correspond histologically to Grade IV.

1.9.4.1.1 Desmoplastic Medulloblastoma (Figs. 61–63)

A variant of medulloblastoma characterized by a dense intercellular network of reticulin fibres and the presence of pale, reticulin-free islands containing typical medulloblastoma cells with neuronal or astrocytic differentiation. Features of incipient neuronal or glial differentiation, if present, are usually restricted to the reticulin-free islands. Macroscopically, this variant may be partially well-defined, with a tendency for superficial location in the lateral lobes of the cerebellum.

Biological behaviour: Some reports suggest a slightly better prognosis for this variant when compared to ordinary medulloblastomas; histologically, the desmoplastic medulloblastoma also corresponds to Grade IV.

1.9.4.1.2 Medullomyoblastoma (Figs. 64, 65)

A very rare variant of medulloblastoma with distinct rhabdomyoblastic differentiation.

This variant contains focal accumulations of striated and, occasionally, non-striated muscle fibres. Myogenic differentiation can be identified by immunoreactivity of portions of the tumour for muscle markers, e.g. desmin, myoglobin and muscle-specific actin.

1.9.4.1.3 Melanotic Medulloblastoma (Fig. 66)

A rare variant of medulloblastoma with foci of epithelial, melanin-containing cells in addition to typical medulloblastoma-like areas. The melanotic cells may form gland-like or papillary structures. Growth and biological behaviour correspond to that of ordinary medulloblastomas. Some authors maintain that this lesion constitutes a cerebral form of the often benign melanotic neuroectodermal tumour of infancy (progonoma), a tumour preferentially involving the maxilla. Melanotic medulloblastomas, in contrast, are highly malignant.

2 Tumours of Cranial and Spinal Nerves

2.1 Schwannoma (Neurilemmoma, Neurinoma) (Figs. 67, 68)

An encapsulated and sometimes cystic tumour composed of spindle-shaped neoplastic Schwann cells.

Two basic histological patterns are seen in most lesions; densely cellular areas composed of compact elongated cells often associated with palisading (Antoni A pattern) and a less cellular, loosely textured pattern in which cells often contain lipid (Antoni B pattern). Hyperchromatic, bizarre nuclei may occur but do not, even in the presence of occasional mitoses, carry a poor prognosis. Tumour cells consistently show immunoreactivity for S-100 protein and Leu 7. Vessels are typically hyalinized and are often surrounded by haemosiderin deposits. Pigmentation, when evident, is usually due to lipofuscin and haemosiderin accumulation, although melanin pigmentation is found in exceptional cases (see Sect. 2.1.3). Axons of the parent nerve are usually found stretched over the tumour capsule rather than being dispersed within its substance.

Although schwannomas may arise on any cranial or spinal nerve, most involve the acoustic nerve or the dorsal roots of spinal nerves. Bilateral acoustic schwannomas are the hallmark of neurofibromatosis type II.

Biological behaviour: Schwannomas correspond histologically to Grade I.

2.1.1 Cellular Schwannoma

A schwannoma characterized by high cellularity, predominance of the Antoni A pattern and the presence of variable mitotic activity. Necrosis may be observed. Essential architectural features of ordinary schwannoma, such as encapsulation and vascular hyalinization, are also present.

2.1.2 Plexiform Schwannoma

A schwannoma composed of racemose worm-like arrangements of tumour cells, aggregated or dispersed in connective tissue. Most are small and usually dermal or subcutaneous. Mitoses may be present in small numbers.

2.1.3 Melanotic Schwannoma (Fig. 69)

A schwannoma in which melanin pigment may be so abundant that it obscures cytological features. Rare examples, accompanied by psammomatous calcification, may be hereditary (Carney triad).

2.2 Neurofibroma (Figs. 70, 71)

A demarcated or, particularly in dermal and subcutaneous tissue, diffuse tumour composed of Schwann cells, fibroblasts and perineurial cells. The lesion varies in cellularity as well as in its content of collagen and mucosubstances.

The cells exhibit wavy nuclear and cellular contours and are disposed singly or in intersecting fascicles. Bizarre nuclei seen in tumours of long standing, are a degenerative feature of no prognostic value. Neurites may be demonstrated in large neoplasms, particularly near proximal and distal margins where transition to normal nerve is seen, or within small tumours wherein fibres are not widely dispersed. Antoni A and B patterns are not seen, but focal palisading (Meissner corpuscles) or tight whorling (Pacinian corpuscles) may be found. Some neurofibromas contain sufficiently dense arrays of Schwann cells to suggest a 'schwannoma in neurofibroma'. Immunoreactivity for S-100 protein and Leu 7 is a regular feature. Mast cells may be conspicuous. Neurofibromas occur as solitary lesions or as a component of neurofibromatosis.

2.2.1 Circumscribed (Solitary) Neurofibroma

A single fusiform or globular neurofibroma, most often unassociated with neurofibromatosis.

2.2.2 Plexiform Neurofibroma (Fig. 72)

A grossly racemose or "bag of worms"-like neurofibroma involving numerous branches of a nerve. Such tumours are often glistening in appearance, due to their high stromal mucus content. Foci of higher cellularity with cytological atypia may be seen. A minor but significant proportion of plexiform neurofibromas undergoes malignant transformation, an event marked by hypercellularity, atypia and brisk mitotic activity.
Note: The term "neuroma" is not used for the above entities (Sects. 2.1, 2.2) since it has been applied to non-neoplastic overgrowths of nerve fibres, Schwann cells and scar tissue that follow trauma, e.g. traumatic neuroma and Morton neuroma.

2.3 Malignant Peripheral Nerve Sheath Tumour (MPNST) (Neurogenic Sarcoma, Neurofibrosarcoma, Anaplastic Neurofibroma,"Malignant Schwannoma") (Fig. 73)

Generally the malignant counterpart of neurofibroma since malignant forms of schwannoma are extremely rare.

Sarcomatous transformation of neurofibromas is a recognized complication, particularly of plexiform tumours in the setting of neurofibromatosis I, wherein either these or solitary tumours may show anaplastic change. Transformation within a lesion is more often uni- or multifocal than generalized. Immunoreactivity for S-100 protein and Leu 7 is usually less than in benign nerve sheath tumours.

Biological behaviour: MPNST and its variants correspond histologically to Grade III or IV.

2.3.1 Epithelioid MPNST (Fig. 74)

A rare form of MPNST composed of plump, often eosinophilic cells with vesicular nuclei and prominent eosinophilic nucleoli. Cells are clustered in such a way as to simulate carcinoma. Immunoreactivity for S-100 protein is often strong.

2.3.2 MPNST with Divergent Mesenchymal and/or Epithelial Differentiation

A malignant nerve sheath tumour exhibiting malignant cartilage, bone, skeletal muscle, and/or mucinous, neuroendocrine or undifferentiated epithelium. Such features are often focal, bear no prognostic significance and occur both within and outside the setting of neurofibromatosis.

2.3.3 Melanotic MPNST

A rare variant of malignant peripheral nerve sheath tumour with melanin-producing tumour cells which may be clustered or diffusely distributed within the neoplasm.

3 Tumours of the Meninges

The classification of this group of tumours is based upon the view that the meninges include the dura, the cap cell (meningothelial) layer of the arachnoid membrane and of arachnoid granulations, as well as subarachnoid blood vessels, fibroblasts and the pia.

3.1 Tumours of Meningothelial Cells

3.1.1 Meningioma

A benign tumour composed of neoplastic meningothelial (arachnoid) cells.

Although most meningiomas are attached to dura, particularly in areas where arachnoid villi are numerous, some occur at unusual sites such as the choroid plexus stroma. Occasional examples arise within cerebral parenchyma, presumably from perivascular arachnoidal cells. Rare meningiomas arise within bone, but the vast majority secondarily invade it, producing either an osteoblastic or, less often, a lytic reaction. Invasion of muscle or soft tissue may also be seen. Most meningiomas are demarcated but unencapsulated; finger-like projections often penetrate surrounding mesenchymal tissues. Occasional tumours, termed "meningioma en-plaque", exhibit carpet-like growth over dural surfaces. Most meningiomas are non-invasive. Microscopically, a number of subtypes are recognized, nearly all of which exhibit vimentin, desmoplakin, EMA and, less often, cytokeratin and S-100 protein immunoreactivity. Although the majority exhibit similar biological behaviour, some variants are associated with unique clinical features.

Biological behaviour: Although meningiomas exhibit a distinct tendency to recurrence, the following variants all correspond histologically to Grade I.

3.1.1.1 Meningothelial Meningioma (Fig. 75)

A tumour consisting of demarcated, solid lobules of meningothelial cells often with ill-defined cell membranes. Nuclei are round to oval, pale and exhibit a tendency to margination of chromatin, thus mimicking nuclear holes. Cytoplasmic invagination and nuclear irregularities commonly produce pseudoinclusions. Perilobular collagen and reticulin deposition is variable. Whorls are not a prominent feature of this type of meningioma. In some examples, large or giant cells with bizarre single or multiple nuclei may be encountered; this feature alone does not signify aggressive behaviour or malignancy. Mitoses are infrequent or absent.

3.1.1.2 Fibrous (Fibroblastic) Meningioma (Fig. 76)

A meningioma in which spindle-shaped cells somewhat resembling fibroblasts predominate. Parallel and interlacing bundles of cells with abundant intercellular collagen and reticulin are distinctive features. Whorl formation and psammoma bodies are infrequent.

3.1.1.3 Transitional (Mixed) Meningioma (Fig. 77)

A meningioma with a mixed pattern or intermediate features, combining those of meningothelial as well as fibrous meningioma. Such tumours show a distinct tendency to concentric whorl formation, often around a central capillary. Some of the whorls contain hyaline, occasionally calcified cores or psammoma bodies.

3.1.1.4 Psammomatous Meningioma (Fig. 78)

A meningioma, often composed of transitionally appearing cells, in which psammoma bodies are abundant. In some examples, only small nests of meningothelial cells may be seen within mineralized areas. Many such tumours are spinal or arise in the olfactory groove.

3.1.1.5 Angiomatous Meningioma (Fig. 79)

A meningioma in which large or small vascular channels are prominent. Intervening nests of meningothelial cells may be inconspicuous. Tumours in which capillary-size vessels are particularly numerous may mimic haemangioblastoma.

3.1.1.6 Microcystic Meningioma (Fig. 80)

A loose-textured meningioma composed of cells with elongated processes circumscribing intercellular microcysts containing pale eosinophilic mucin. Pleomorphic and hyperchromatic nuclei often contain cytoplasmic inclusions. Eosinophilic, periodic acid-Schiff (PAS)-positive globules, as are seen in secretory meningioma (see Sect. 3.1.1.7), may also be observed. As a rule, whorls and psammoma bodies are scant or absent.

3.1.1.7 Secretory Meningioma (Figs. 81, 82)

A meningioma with meningothelial or transitional features which shows epithelial differentiation as evidenced by the presence of glandular lumina, one or more of which may be seen within a cell. The lumina contain eosinophilic, strongly PAS-positive globules which are immunoreactive for CEA and secretory component. Immediately surrounding cells are strongly cytokeratin-positive.

3.1.1.8 Clear Cell Meningioma (Fig. 83)

An often patternless meningioma composed of closely apposed polygonal cells with clear, glycogen-rich (PAS-positive, diastaselabile) cytoplasm. Whorl formation is vague at best. Psammoma bodies are often lacking. Such tumours show a proclivity for the cerebellopontine angle and the cauda equina region.

3.1.1.9 Chordoid Meningioma (Fig. 84)

A meningioma which exhibits lobularity and a tendency to form chains of eosinophilic, occasionally vacuolated cells and thus mimics chordoma. Interlobular stroma may contain a lymphoplasmacytic infiltrate. Such tumours usually show focal meningothelial or transitional features. Cytokeratin, S-100 protein and even EMA are usually less positive than in chordomas. Psammoma bodies are few in number. Polyclonal gammopathy and/or anaemia may be associated with this tumour or its recurrence.

3.1.1.10 Lymphoplasmacyte-rich Meningioma (Fig. 85)

A meningioma (of meningothelial, transitional or even fibrous type) with dense lymphoplasmacytic infiltrates, which may be present to such an extent that they obscure the underlying meningioma pattern. Polyclonal gammopathy and/or anaemia may be associated with this tumour or its recurrence.

3.1.1.11 Metaplastic Meningioma

Meningiomas, usually of meningothelial, transitional or fibrous type which show metaplasia to xanthomatous, cartilaginous, osseous, myxoid or lipomatous cells.

3.1.2 Atypical Meningioma (Figs. 86, 87)

Meningiomas in which several of the following features are evident: frequent mitoses, increased cellularity, small cells with high nuclear cytoplasmic ratios and/or prominent nucleoli, uninterrupted patternless or sheet-like growth and foci of "spontaneous" or geographic necrosis.

Nuclear atypia alone or simply invasion of dura or bone does not qualify a tumour for the designation "atypical".

Biological behaviour: Atypical meningiomas show an increased tendency to recurrence and correspond histologically to Grade II.

3.1.3 Papillary Meningioma (Fig. 88)

An aggressive highly cellular meningioma composed, in part, of perivascular pseudopapillae.

The nuclei are monotonous and resemble those of meningothelial cells, particularly in areas wherein the growth pattern is that of a more ordinary meningioma. Cells terminating on the vasculature of papillae exhibit tapering processes similar to those of pseudorosettes in ependymomas. Intercellular reticulin may be noted. Whorls and psammoma bodies are generally lacking in papillary areas. Mitoses are present but vary in number. Like typical meningiomas, most papillary meningiomas are immunoreactive for EMA and may express cytokeratin and S-100 reactivity as well. These reactivities usually diminish with increasing anaplasia. Papillary meningiomas most commonly occur in young patients.

Biological behaviour: Papillary meningiomas are often aggressive, undergoing frequent recurrence, brain invasion and late metastasis. They correspond histologically to Grade II or III.

3.1.4 Anaplastic (Malignant) Meningioma (Fig. 89)

A meningioma exhibiting histological features of frank malignancy far in excess of the abnormalities noted in atypical meningioma. These include obviously malignant cytology, a high mitotic index and conspicuous necrosis.

Meningiomas showing transition to anaplastic collagen-producing spindle cells have been loosely termed 'sarcomatous meningioma', a term not endorsed by the working group. Some participants maintained that gross brain invasion, not only metastasis, qualifies a tumour for the designation malignant; such lesions do not invariably exhibit histological malignancy and their immunocytochemical features may be similar to those of ordinary meningiomas.

Biological behaviour: Anaplastic meningiomas correspond histologically to Grade III.

3.2 Mesenchymal, Non-meningothelial Tumours

The nomenclature and definition of these tumours follow that of the WHO "*Histological Typing of Soft Tissue Tumours*".

Benign Neoplasms

3.2.1 Osteocartilaginous Tumours

Chondroma, osteochondroma and osteoma form solitary masses composed of varying proportions of chondrocytes and osteocytes showing little or no atypia. Most are meningeal, the dura being involved more often than the leptomeninges. Rare examples involving choroid plexus stroma and brain parenchyma have been reported.

3.2.2 Lipoma

A mass of fully differentiated adipose tissue, with or without a minor component of fibrous or vascular tissue.

A cytologically benign lesion, usually lying in the midline, e.g. related to the corpus callosum, third ventricle and quadrigeminal region, the intraspinal space or, less often, in other locations such as the Sylvian fissure or the cerebellopontine angle. Intraspinal lipomas are most often leptomeningeal. In some cases a malformative basis is implied by the finding of Schwann cells, bone or cartilage, or by an accompanying developmental abnormality such as absence of the corpus callosum. Vascular examples, loosely termed "angiolipoma" have also been described; almost all involve spinal epidural soft tissues.

3.2.3 Fibrous Histiocytoma

A firm circumscribed mass composed of a mixture of fibroblasts as well as histiocyte-like cells disposed in a storiform pattern and associated with a delicate or well-formed collagenous stroma.

The proportions of fibrous and histiocyte-like cells vary considerably. Foam cells, siderophages, Touton giant cells and lymphocytes may also be observed. Pleomorphism is minimal as is mitotic activity. Areas of collagenous sclerosis or myxoid change may be seen.

3.2.4 Others

A number of benign mesenchymal neoplasms may rarely affect the CNS. Among others, these include fibroma, leiomyoma, rhabdomyoma, glomangioma, epithelioid haemangioendothelioma and myxoma.

Malignant Neoplasms

3.2.5 Haemangiopericytoma (Figs. 90, 91)

A monotonous cellular tumour composed of plump or polygonal cells with oval nuclei and scant, ill-defined cytoplasm accompanied by an often dense intercellular pattern of reticulin staining, typically surrounding vascular spaces lined by normal endothelium.

The reticulin corresponds to the production, by tumour cells, of an amorphous basement-membrane-like material. The differentiation of tumour cells varies from pericytic to myoid and fibroblastic. As a result, some examples exhibit more elongated cells accompanied by considerable intercellular collagen. The cellularity of the tumour is often interrupted by characteristic "staghorn" vascular spaces as well as patches of hypocellularity and sclerosis. Mitoses vary from few to numerous. Necrosis is uncommon. Papillae formation, tight whorls and psammoma bodies are not observed. Haemangiopericytomas are vimentin-positive but, unlike meningiomas, they lack EMA reactivity. Occasional tumours show reactivity for desmin or muscle-specific actin.

Biological behaviour: Since haemangiopericytomas show a strong tendency for recurrence and metastasis, they are generally regarded as malignant neoplasms; however, some haemangiopericytomas are associated with a less aggressive behaviour. They correspond histologically to Grade II or III.

3.2.6 Chondrosarcoma

A tumour composed of cytologically malignant chondrocytes.

Most involve the dura and resemble chondrosarcoma of bone and soft tissues. Examples with myxoid features have been termed "chordoid sarcoma". Unlike chordoma, the principal differential diagnostic consideration of midline chondrosarcomas, chondrosarcoma lacks cytokeratin and epithelial membrane reactivity; vimentin and S-100 positively are common to both tumours.

3.2.6.1 Mesenchymal Chondrosarcoma

A tumour composed of sheets of light microscopically undifferentiated small cells punctuated by islands of atypical to malignant hyaline cartilage. The small cell component may exhibit a growth pattern similar to haemangiopericytoma. Intercellular reticulin staining is variable. Most mesenchymal chondrosarcomas arise in the dura, but parenchymal examples have been described. Recurrence is frequent and systemic metastases may occur.

3.2.7 Malignant Fibrous Histiocytoma

A tumour composed of cytologically malignant fibroblasts, myofibroblasts, histiocyte-like and undifferentiated cells.

These uncommon, aggressive tumours vary in their composition of spindle cells (fibroblasts and myofibroblasts) and pleomorphic, sometimes lipidized giant cells. Mitoses are readily identified and necrosis may be observed. Somewhat arbitrarily, tumours composed predominantly of spindle cells or histiocyte-like cells have been designated fibrosarcoma and malignant fibrous histiocytoma, respectively. Their morphology is identical to that of soft tissue tumours of the same type. Despite the immunohistochemical demonstration of α_1-antitrypsin in many examples, more specific histiocytic markers are negative. Malignant fibrous histiocytomas react for vimentin but lack desmin and S-100 reactivity. Lesions may be either meningeal or parenchymal in origin. Malignant fibrous or fibrohistiocytic elements often comprise the mesenchymal component of gliosarcomas (see Sect. 1.1.3.2).

3.2.8 Rhabdomyosarcoma

A malignant tumour composed of neoplastic rhabdomyoblasts.

The predominant variant of this rare tumour in the central nervous system is the "embryonal" subtype. Microscopically, it resembles the same lesion occurring in soft tissues. The small round tumour cells possess eccentric eosinophilic cytoplasm which is often fibril-rich. Cross striations may be difficult to find, except in tumours with strap-shaped cells or myotubes. Mitoses are present. Immunocytochemistry shows positivity for vimentin and, in most cases, desmin, myoglobin, or muscle-specific actin. This lesion often occurs within brain parenchyma without an associatiated meningeal component.

3.2.9 Meningeal Sarcomatosis

A sarcoma arising from and diffusely infiltrating the meninges.

Grossly, these may appear multifocal or as contiguous, widespread infiltrates. The poorly differentiated cells are usually round to fusiform in shape and possess scant cytoplasm. Mitoses are present but vary in number. Immunochemistry is required to exclude malignant gliomas, embryonal tumours of the CNS including primitive PNETs, small cell sarcomas of other type and even lymphomas.

3.2.10 Others

A variety of sarcomas may, on rare occasions, affect the CNS; these include fibrosarcoma, osteosarcoma, leiomyosarcoma, Ewing sarcoma, rhabdoid tumour, angiosarcoma and liposarcoma. In addition, tumours without light microscopic, immunohistochemical or ultrastructurally distinct features also fall into this category. Such tumours may be regarded as "undifferentiated sarcoma".

3.3 Primary Melanocytic Lesions

These neoplasms vary from benign to malignant and from diffuse to nodular. With the exception of melanocytoma, approximately 25% are associated with the neurocutaneous melanosis syndrome. Melanotic lesions show immunoreactivity for S-100 protein, HMB-45 and vimentin.

3.3.1 Diffuse Melanosis

A cytologically benign, diffuse proliferation of melanocytes involving the leptomeninges.

This proliferation is diffuse in nature, and may involve brain parenchyma by extending into perivascular (Virchow-Robin) spaces.

3.3.2 Melanocytoma (Fig. 92)

A nodular, usually leptomeningeal tumour composed of uniform neoplastic melanocytes with vesicular nuclei and variable, often dense cytoplasmic melanin content.

Tumour cells may possess prominent nucleoli but show little or no mitotic activity. These benign lesions frequently arise in the thoracic spinal region, and less often in the intracranial space where basal structures are usually involved, e.g. Meckel cave. Macrosopically, melanocytomas are grossly black. Although recurrence may be seen, malignant transformation is rare.

3.3.3 Malignant Melanoma

A tumour composed of malignant melanocytes which vary in pigmentation from dense to amelanotic.

Cytologic atypia and mitotic activity are highly variable. Necrosis may be widespread, sparing only perivascular cuffs of viable tumour cells. Such tumours may or may not exhibit diffuse parenchymal and leptomeningeal spread.

3.3.3.1 Meningeal Melanomatosis

A tumour characterized by widespread, diffuse infiltration of the leptomeninges by malignant melanocytes. Associated nodular growth may also occur. This lesion may occur in association with neurocutaneous melanosis.

3.4 Tumours of Uncertain Histogenesis

3.4.1 Haemangioblastoma (Capillary Haemangioblastoma) (Figs. 93, 94)

A well-demarcated, highly vascular and occasionally multifocal tumour that often has an associated cyst and typically connects with the leptomeninges.

The principal or "stromal" cells possess round to somewhat irregular nuclei which tend to be hyperchromatic and have inconspicuous nucleoli. Their eosinophilic and variably lipid-rich cytoplasm is often ill-defined. The cells are uniformly distributed within an intricate network of capillaries (reticular variant) or are clustered, forming large groups circumferentially delimited by capillaries (cellular variant). Glycogen is often abundant. Mitoses are absent or infrequent. Since stromal cells can produce erythropoietin, extramedullary erythropoiesis may be seen within the tumour. Stromal cells are vimentin and neuron-specific enolase positive, may show some GFAP expression, but are negative for EMA. Astrocytic reaction within and at the periphery of the tumours may be striking. The major differential diagnostic consideration is renal cell carcinoma (a feature of von Hippel-Lindau disease), which shows greater clearing of cytoplasm by glycogen, regimentation of cells in geometric patterns and EMA immunoreactivity.

The cerebellum is most often involved. The medulla and spinal cord are alternative sites. Involvement of the cerebral meninges is rare. A small proportion of meningeal haemangioblastomas are associated with von Hippel-Lindau disease, where they may be multiple.

4 Lymphomas and Haemopoietic Neoplasms

4.1 Malignant Lymphomas

Histologically, CNS lymphomas resemble systemic lymphomas; they are almost exclusively non-Hodgkin lymphomas, with a diffuse rather than a follicular/nodular growth pattern. Primary malignant lymphomas of the CNS occur both sporadically and in the setting of immunosuppression, e.g. in patients with the acquired immune deficiency syndrome (AIDS). Preceding or concurrent ocular involvement is noted in some cases. In approximately 10% of cases, foci of systemic spread are noted post-mortem. The intraparenchymal localization of most primary lymphomas contrasts with the typically meningeal localization of lymphoma metastatic to the CNS. Primary lesions are usually deep-seated, often subependymal, and may be bilaterally symmetrical. They may be either solitary or multiple. Those associated with immunosuppression, particularly AIDS, are more likely to be multiple and to exhibit widespread necrosis. Local recurrences and ventricular seeding via the CSF are frequent.

Most primary CNS lymphomas are monoclonal B-cell lesions of the large cell or immunoblastic type. T cell lymphomas are rare. They can be classified according to the NCI Working Formulation (Table 1) or the Kiel classification (Table 2).

Table 1. Non-Hodgkin lymphomas: NCI Working Formulation

Low grade

A. Malignant lymphoma
Small lymphocytic
Consistent with CLL

Clear cell
B. Malignant lymphoma, follicular
Predominantly small cleaved cell
component
Diffuse areas
Sclerosis
C. Malignant lymphoma, follicular
Mixed, small cleaved and large cell
Diffuse areas
Sclerosis

Intermediate grade

D. Malignant lymphoma, follicular
Predominantly large cell
Diffuse areas
plasmacytoma
Sclerosis
E. Malignant lymphoma, diffuse
Small cleaved cell
Sclerosis
F. Malignant lymphoma, diffuse
Mixed, small and large cell
Sclerosis
Epithelioid cell component
G. Malignant lymphoma, diffuse
Large cell
Cleaved cell
Non-cleaved cell
Sclerosis

High grade

H. Malignant lymphoma
Large cell, immunoblastic
Plasmacytoid
Plasmacytoid

Polymorphous
Epithelioid cell

I. Malignant lymphoma
Lymphoblastic
Convoluted cell
Non-convoluted cell
J. Malignant lymphoma
Small non-cleaved cell
Burkitt's
Follicular areas

Miscellaneous
Composite
Mycosis fungoides
Histiocytic
Extramedullary

Unclassifiable
Other

From Cancer 49: 2112-2135, 1982

Table 2. Non-Hodgkin lymphomas — Updated Kiel classification[1]

B-cell	T-cell
Low-grade malignant lymphomas	
Lymphocytic Chronic lymphocytic leukaemia Prolymphocytic leukaemia Hairy-cell leukaemia	Lymphocytic Chronic lymphocytic leukaemia Prolymphocytic leukaemia
	Small cell, cerebriform Mycosis fungoides, Sezary's syndrome
Lymphoplasmacytic /-cytoid (immunocytoma)	Lymphoepithelioid (Lennert's lymphoma)
Plasmacytic	Angioimmunoblastic (AILD, LgX)
Centroblastic-centrocytic follicular ± diffuse diffuse	T-zone lymphoma
Centrocytic	Pleomorphic, small cell (HTLV-I±)
Monocytoid	
High-grade malignant lymphomas	
Centroblastic	Pleomorphic, medium-sized and large cell (HTLV-I±)
Immunoblastic	Immunoblastic (HTLV-I±)
Large cell, anaplastic (Ki-1+)	Large cell, anaplastic (Ki-1+)
Burkitt lymphoma	
Lymphoblastic	Lymphoblastic
Rare types	*Rare types*

[1] Lennert K, Feller AC (1991) Histopathology of non-Hodgkin-lymphomas (according to the updated Kiel classification), 2nd edn., Springer, Berlin Heidelberg New York

Hodgkin disease very rarely affects the CNS as a primary neoplasm.

4.2 Plasmacytoma

A tumour composed of mature-appearing neoplastic plasma cells.

The skull and the intracranial dura are common sites of plasmacytoma. Monoclonal globulin production is a diagnostic feature. Some lesions are precursors of multiple myeloma.

4.3 Granulocytic Sarcoma

A tumour composed of variably differentiated neoplastic granulocytes.

The lesion precedes or is concurrent with, acute myelogenous leukemia. Most are subdural.

4.4 Others

5 Germ Cell Tumours

Primary intracranial germ cell tumours occur principally in the pineal and suprasellar regions. Some, particularly germinomas, may also arise in the thalamus or basal ganglia. Males, usually children or young adults, are more often affected. The classification and features of these tumours are the same as are described in the WHO *Histological Typing of Testis Tumours*.

5.1 Germinoma (Fig. 95)

Histopathologically identical to the testicular seminoma, the germinoma is composed of uniform cells resembling primitive germ cells. Large vesicular nuclei, prominent nucleoli and clear or pale, glycogen-rich cytoplasm are typical features. Scattered human chrorionic gonadotropin (HCG)-positive, syncytiotrophoblastic giant cells are common, but prognostically unimportant. Germinomas are immunoreactive for placental alkaline phosphatase. Lymphocytes and granulomatous infiltrates are usually present and may mask the underlying neoplasm.

5.2 **Embryonal Carcinoma** (Fig. 96)

A tumour composed of cells of primitive epithelial appearance, sometimes with clear cytoplasm, growing in a variety of patterns, including solid sheets or poorly formed glands. The tumour is highly mitotically active and often shows foci of necrosis.

5.3 **Yolk Sac Tumour (Endodermal Sinus Tumour)** (Figs. 97, 98)

A tumour composed of primitive appearing cells, typically growing in a loosely knit or reticular network. Tubular, papillary and solid patterns may also be present. Eosinophilic intracytoplasmic or stromal globules containing α-fetoprotein are a diagnostic feature.

5.4 **Choriocarcinoma**

A highly malignant tumour composed of both syncytiotrophoblast and cytotrophoblast, arranged in a characteristic bilayered pattern. Immunoreactivity for HCG is strong.

5.5 **Teratoma**

A tumour composed of an admixture of different tissue types representative of ectoderm, endoderm and mesoderm. Accordingly, the immunoreactivity of teratomas is that of the various component tissues.

5.5.1 **Immature Teratoma** (Fig. 99)

A teratoma composed of incompletely differentiated tissues resembling those of the fetus. Mitoses are typically present.

5.5.2 **Mature Teratoma** (Fig. 100)

A teratoma composed exclusively of fully differentiated tissues, sometimes arranged in such a manner as to resemble normal tissue relationships. Mitoses are absent or rare.

5.5.3 **Teratoma with Malignant Transformation**

A rare form of teratoma containing malignant components of the type typically encountered in other organs and tissues. Sarcomas of various type, or epithelial malignancies such as squamous cell or adenocarcinoma are most common.

5.6 Mixed Germ Cell Tumours

Any combination of the above mentioned histological types may occur. Germinoma is frequently combined with other germ cell tumours. The so-called teratocarcinoma consists of a combination of embryonal carcinoma and immature teratoma.

6 Cysts and Tumour-like Lesions

6.1 Rathke Cleft Cyst (Fig. 101)

An intra- or suprasellar cyst lined by ciliated, cuboidal to columnar epithelium, goblet cells and occasional pituitary endocrine cells. These are the same elements lining the small cysts and glands found normally between the anterior and posterior lobes.

6.2 Epidermoid Cyst

Thin-walled and "pearly", these cysts are lined by a delicate layer of keratin-producing squamous epithelial cells containing keratohyalin granules. The underlying stroma is scant. Epidermoid cysts occur throughout the neuraxis, the most common sites being the skull and cerebellopontine angle. "Cholesteatoma" and "pearly tumour" are synonyms occasionally used for this lesion. Malignant transformation is rare.

6.3 Dermoid Cyst

A cyst lined by squamous epithelium with underlying dermal appendages, including hair follicles and adnexae. Dermoid cysts frequently occur in the midline and may communicate via a sinus tract to the cutaneous surface. Their sebaceous contents are greasy or cheesy and often contain hair. The underlying "dermal" stroma is more abundant than in epidermoid cysts. Malignant transformation is extremely rare.

6.4 Colloid Cyst of the Third Ventricle (Fig. 102)

A cyst occurring in the anterior third ventricle near the foramen of Monro. The lesion is lined by cuboidal to columnar, ciliated and/or goblet cells which may become flattened and atrophic under pressure. Capsular stroma is scant. Superimposed xanthogranulomatous change may be noted. Since these cysts are endodermal in nature, the terms 'paraphyseal cyst' and 'neuro-epithelial cyst' are misnomers.

6.5 Enterogenous Cyst

A cyst lined by mucin-secreting and/or ciliated, cuboidal to columnar epithelium resembling that of the respiratory and intestinal tracts. Most examples are intradural, where some are connected by an anterior defect in the dura to an adjacent vertebral body.

6.6 Neuroglial Cyst

A cyst lined either by ependyma or, less specifically, by reactive astrocytes.

6.7 Granular Cell Tumour (Choristoma, Pituicytoma) (Fig. 103)

An intra- or suprasellar neoplasm composed of finely granular cells similar to those occurring incidentally as clusters and 'tumourlets' in the normal pituitary stalk and posterior pituitary. This lysosome-rich, astrocyte-derived tumour is not related to the granular tumour of soft tissue.

6.8 Hypothalamic Neuronal Hamartoma (Fig. 104)

A non-neoplastic mass of hypothalamic tissue composed of mature and often clustered, neurons and a minor glial stroma. Most of these lesions occur at the base of the brain and are attached to the floor of the third ventricle or to a posterior communicating artery. Large examples may deeply indent the third ventricle. Some examples secrete hypothalamic hormones and produce endocrine symptoms.

6.9 Nasal Glial Heterotopia

A congenitally displaced mass of neuroglial tissue in the nose or paranasal region. Its architecture may be haphazard or well-organized, including grey and white matter in association with leptomeninges and meningeal melanocytes. Some heterotopias communicate with the brain through a defect in the skull and dura (encephalocoele).

6.10 Plasma Cell Granuloma

An inflammatory pseudotumour composed of chronic inflammatory cells among which plasma cells producing polyclonal immunoglobulins predominate. The lesions are usually dura-based and grossly resemble meningiomas.

7 Tumours of the Sellar Region

7.1 Pituitary Adenoma

A benign tumour composed of secretory cells of the adenohypophysis.

Most functional tumours produce prolactin, growth hormone, adrenocorticotropic hormone, thyrotropic hormone or alpha subunit, either singly or in combination. Nonfunctioning tumours often produce either or both luteinizing and follicle-stimulating hormone and/or alpha subunit, or lack hormone content ("null cell adenoma"). Cytologic atypia, low mitotic activity and contiguous invasion of soft tissue and bone may be seen.

7.2 Pituitary Carcinoma

A malignant tumour composed of secretory cells of the adenohypophysis.

Both endocrinologically functional and nonfunctional tumours occur. Pituitary carcinomas exhibit either brain invasion or metastasis. The latter includes discontinuous spread in the cerebrospinal axis or secondary deposits in brain or at extracranial sites such as bone, liver, lung or lymph nodes. Pituitary carcinomas often, but not invariably, show inordinate cytological atypia or mitotic activity.

7.3 Craniopharyngioma

A benign epithelial tumour of the sellar region or the third ventricle presumably derived from remnants of the pituitary anlage.

7.3.1 Adamantinomatous Craniopharyngioma (Fig. 105)

A complex supra and/or intrasellar, cystic epithelial neoplasm containing ribbons, cords and trabeculae of epithelium. Peripheral palisading of nuclei, loose arrangements of squamous cells and nodules of 'wet keratin' are prominent features. Cholesterol clefts, dystrophic calcification, extensive fibrosis and a content of brown cholesterol-containing "machinery oil"-like fluid are typical features.

7.3.2 Papillary Craniopharyngioma (Fig. 106)

A solid or cystic mass, generally uncalcified, consisting of well-differentiated squamous epithelium in sheets which separate to form pseudopapillae. Prominent cellular palisading, cholesterol deposits, fibrosis and "machinery oil" content are lacking. This less frequent form of craniopharyngioma is uncommon in children and often involves the third ventricle.

Biological behaviour: Craniopharyngiomas correspond histologically to Grade I but tend to recur locally. The papillary variant carries a better prognosis.

8 Local Extensions from Regional Tumours

8.1 Paraganglioma (Chemodectoma)

A neuroendocrine tumour composed principally of pale "chief" cells arranged in nests and lobules surrounded by flattened sustentacular cells.

Intracranial (middle ear, glomus jugulare) and spinal (cauda equina region, see Sect. 1.7.8) paragangliomas are most common. The tumours compress rather than invade surrounding structures. They are described in the WHO *Histological Typing of Endocrine Tumours* and *Histological Typing of Tumours of the Upper Respiratory Tract.*

8.2 Chordoma

A tumour of notochordal origin composed of lobular masses of pleomorphic vacuolated cells in a mucoid or myxoid matrix.

Highly vacuolated or "physaliphorous cells" are a typical feature. Cartilage formation may be observed ("chondroid chordoma"). Most examples arise from the clivus or the sacrum. See Sect. 3.2.6 regarding differentiation from chondrosarcoma. Chordomas are defined and discussed in the WHO *Histological Typing of Bone Tumours* and *Histological Typing of Tumours of the Upper Respiratory Tract.*

8.3 Chondroma and Chondrosarcoma

These tumours typically arise from the dura and/or adjacent skull. They are defined and discussed in the WHO *Histological Typing of Bone Tumours*.

8.4 Carcinoma

Carcinomas arising in extracranial tissues may, by extension through skull, spine or soft tissues, impinge on the central nervous system. Some, such as adenoid cystic carcinoma (cylindroma), extend principally along nerves. Other carcinomas, such as prostate cancer, are more likely to extend from metastatic foci in adjacent bone. Neuroendocrine carcinomas of the nose or nasopharynx may extend superiorly to displace or invade the brain.

9 Metastatic Tumours

10 Unclassified Tumours

Tumours that cannot be placed in any of the above categories.

Unless otherwise stated, all the preparations shown in the photomicrographs on the following pages were stained with haematoxylin and eosin.

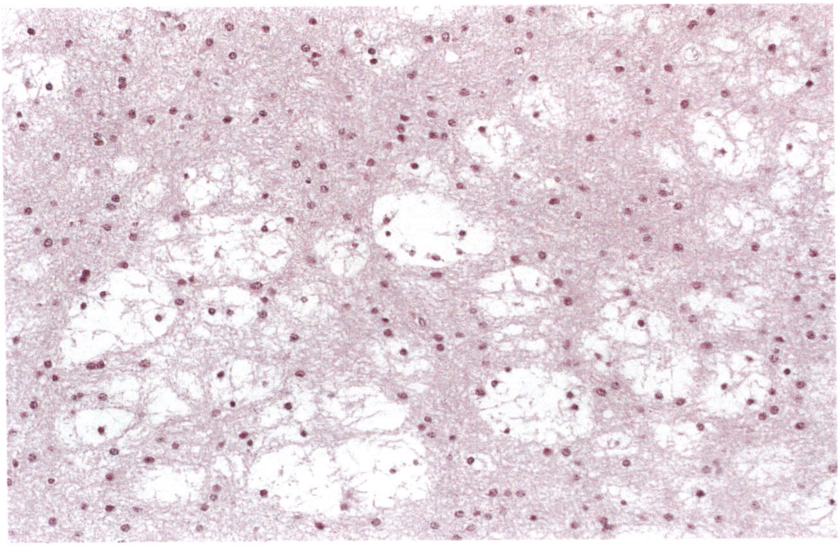

Fig. 1. *Fibrillary astrocytoma* with low cellularity and microcyst formation

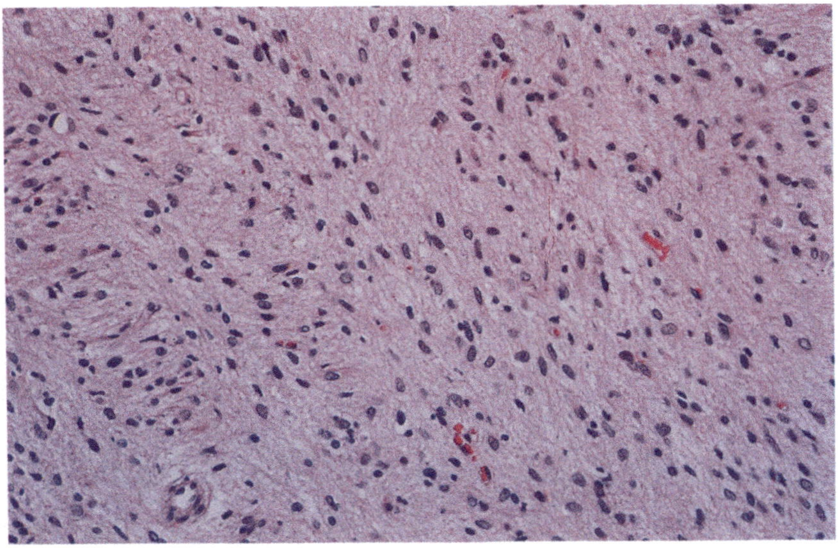

Fig. 2. *Fibrillary astrocytoma* with elongated hyperchromatic nuclei and diffuse infiltration of the white matter

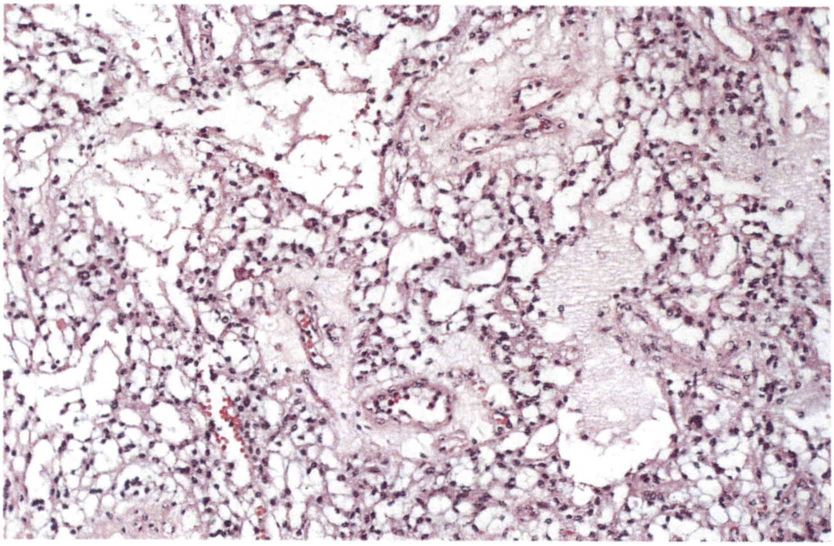

Fig.3. *Protoplasmic astrocytoma.* Small neoplastic astrocytes with scant processes and extensive microcyst formation

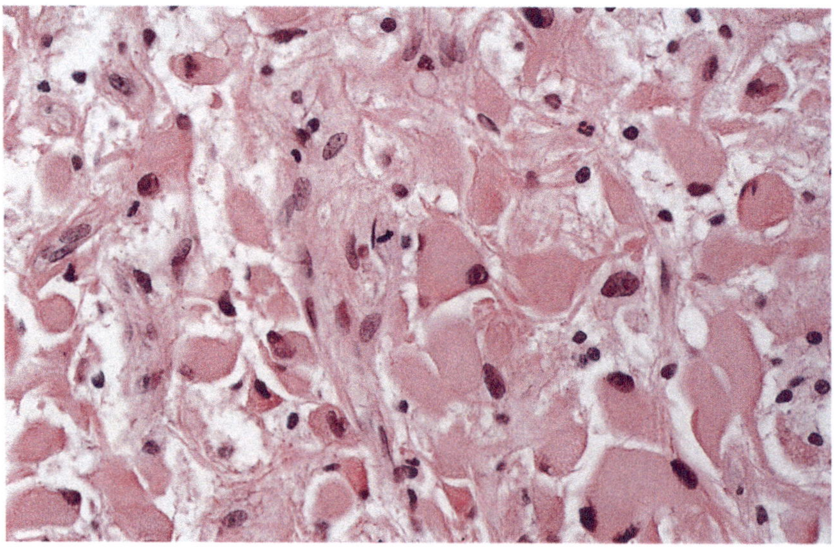

Fig.4. *Gemistocytic astrocytoma.* Large eosinophilic tumour cells with plump processes, eccentric nuclei and occasional mitoses

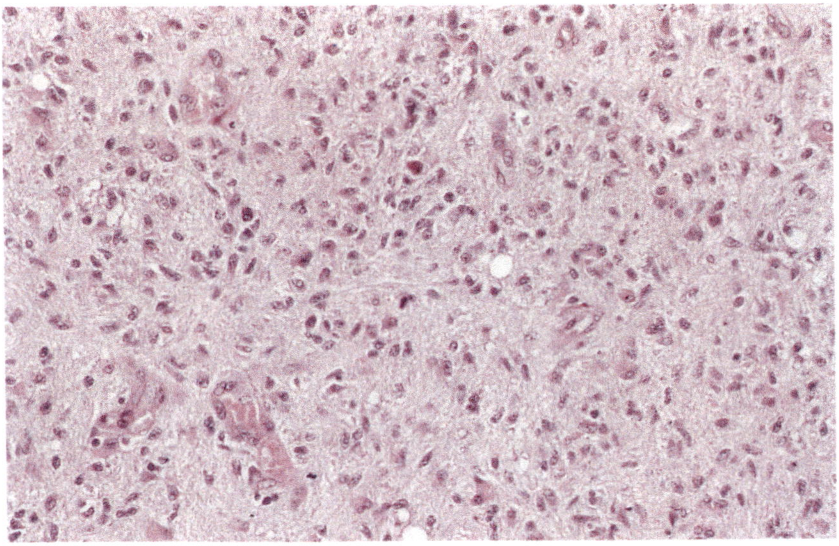

Fig.5. *Anaplastic astrocytoma* with nuclear atypia, frequent mitoses and incipient vascular proliferation

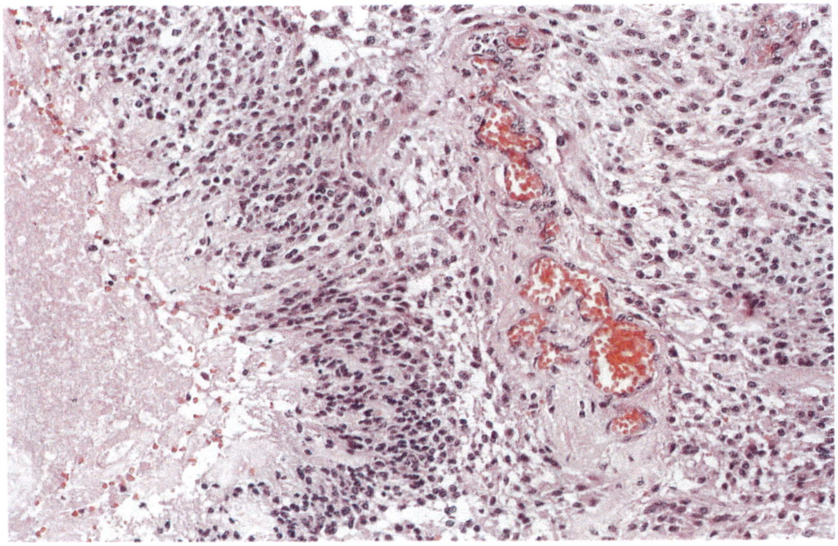

Fig.6. *Glioblastoma*. Small, anaplastic tumour cells, vascular proliferation, and extensive areas of necrosis with pseudopalisading of tumour cells

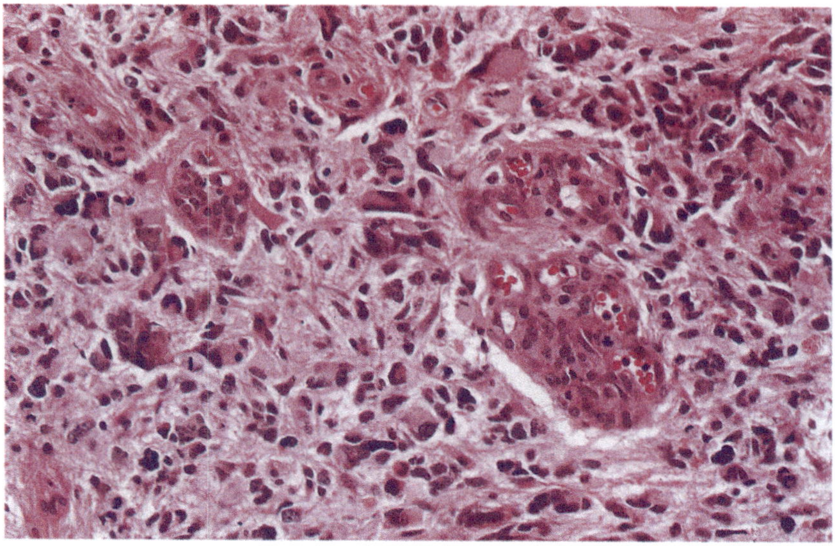

Fig. 7. *Glioblastoma* with glomeruloid vascular proliferation

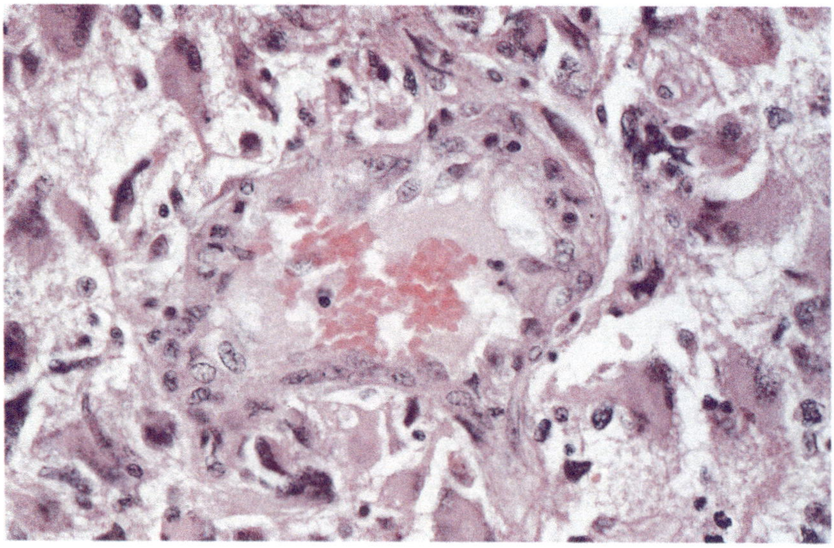

Fig. 8. *Glioblastoma* with marked cellular anaplasia and excessive multi-layered endothelial proliferation

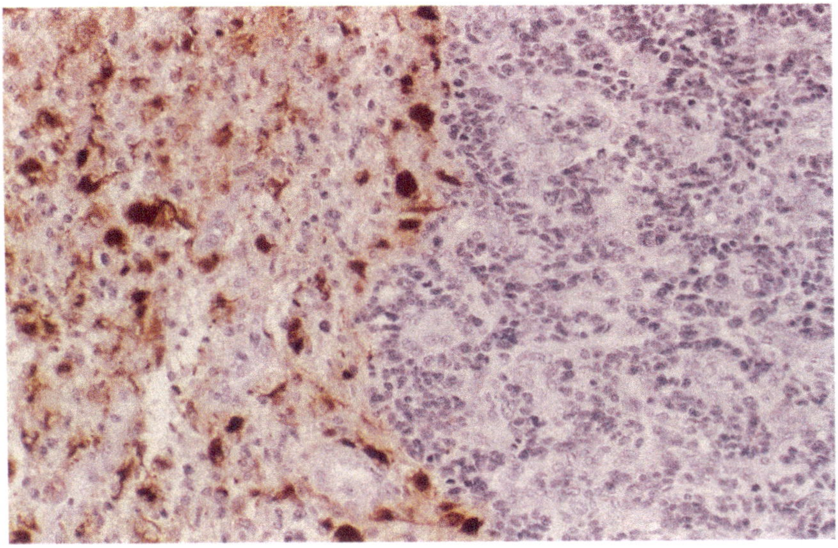

Fig.9. *Glioblastoma.* Sharply delineated anaplastic focus (right) lacking GFAP immunoreactivity

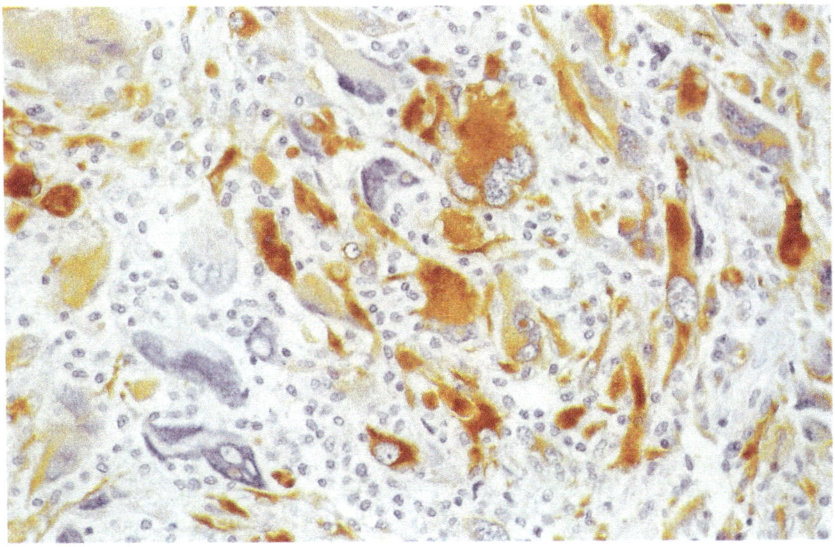

Fig.10. *Giant cell glioblastoma.* Bizarre, often multinucleated giant cells with variable GFAP expression

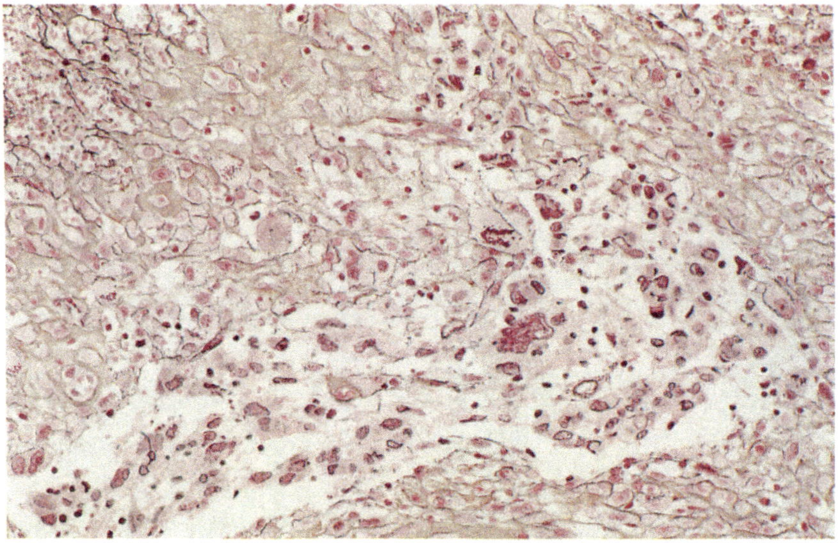

Fig. 11. *Gliosarcoma*. Highly polymorphic neoplastic astrocytes are surrounded by sarcomatous cells which form a dense reticulin network

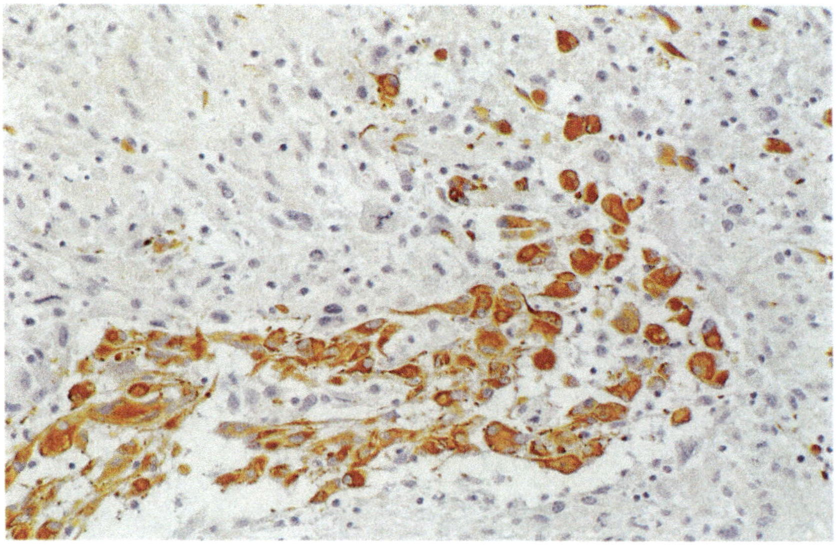

Fig. 12. *Gliosarcoma*. Glial component with marked immunoreactivity for GFAP. Same case and same area as Fig. 11

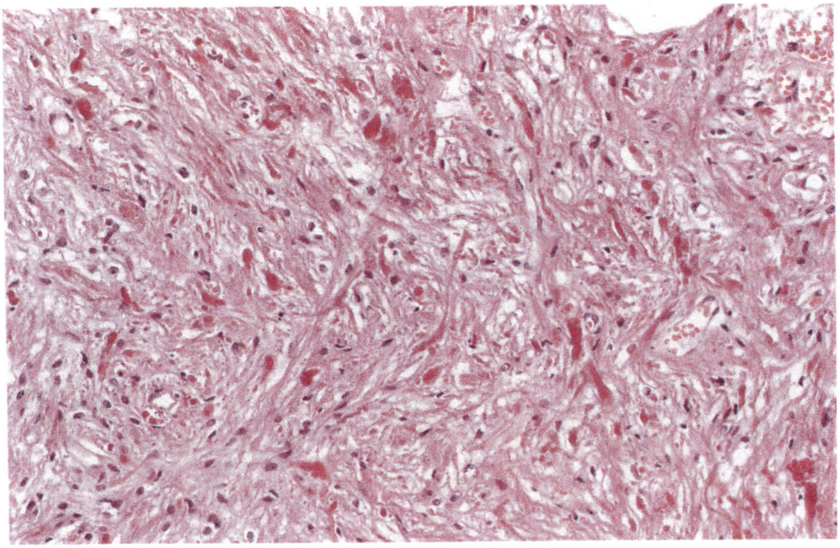

Fig. 13. *Pilocytic astrocytoma*. Elongated, bipolar tumour cells form a dense fibrillary matrix with numerous Rosenthal fibres

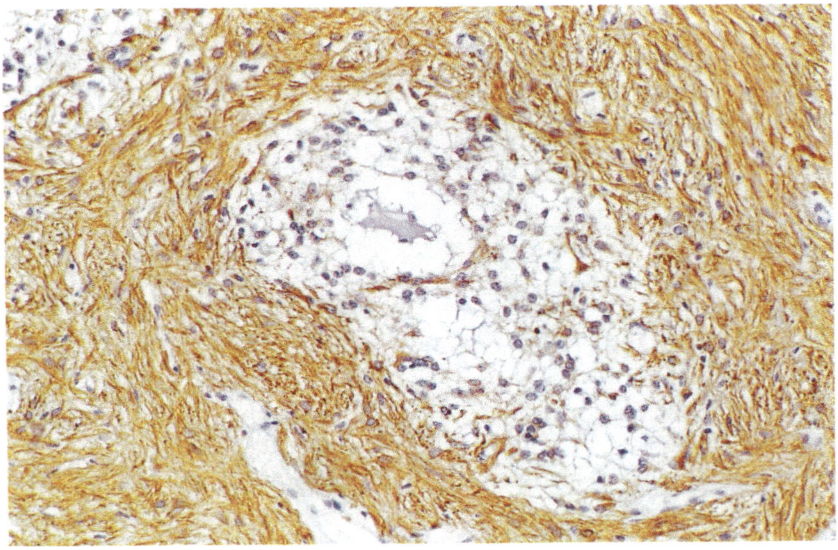

Fig. 14. *Pilocytic astrocytoma*. Biphasic pattern with fibrillary component expressing GFAP and loosely structured areas composed of cells resembling protoplasmic astrocytes which lack GFAP expression and often form microcysts

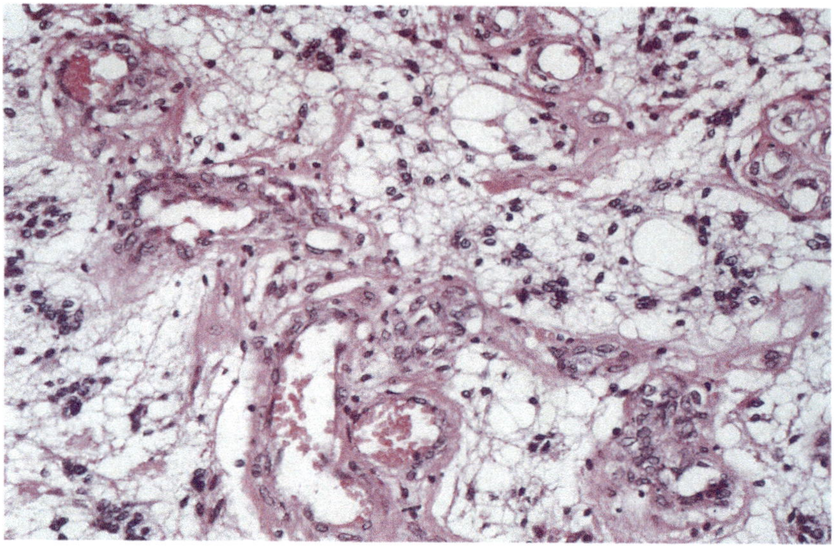

Fig. 15. *Pilocytic astrocytoma*. Marked vascular endothelilal proliferation does not signify malignant behaviour

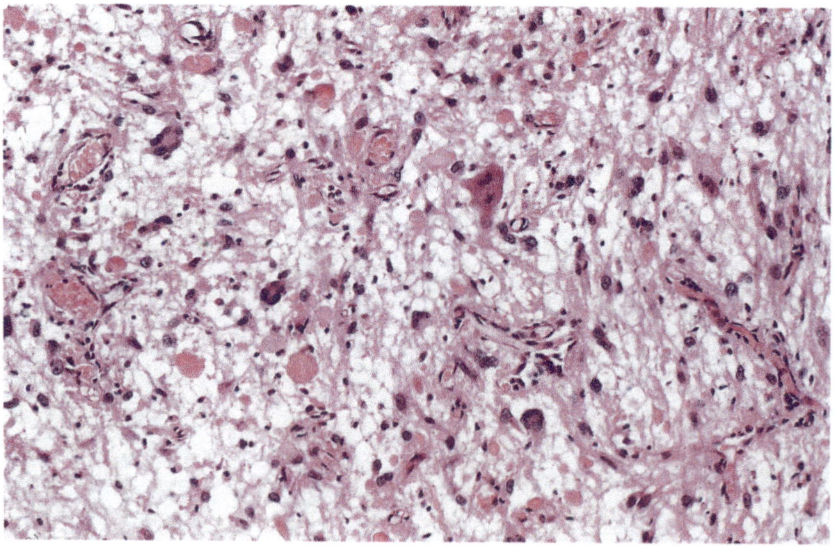

Fig. 16. *Pilocytic astrocytoma*. Marked nuclear atypia and numerous eosinophilic protein droplets

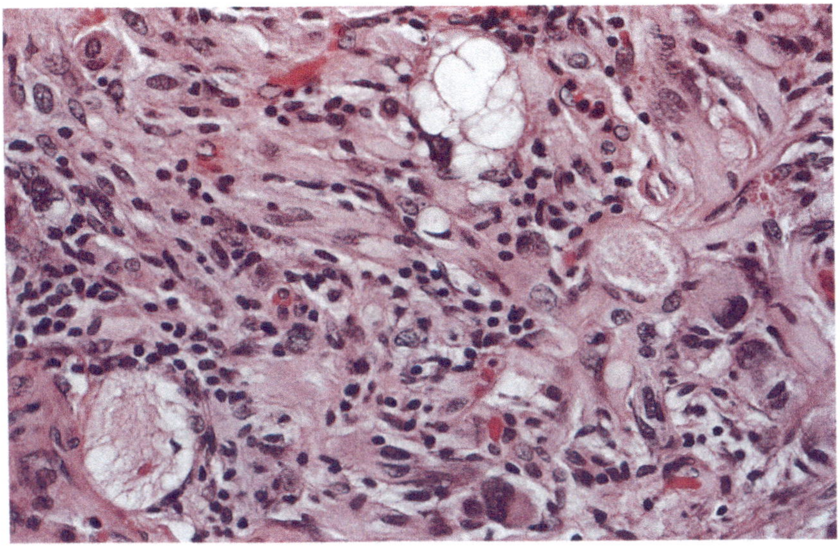

Fig. 17. *Pleomorphic xanthoastrocytoma.* Mixture of small and pleomorphic tumor cells which often contain lipid vacuoles

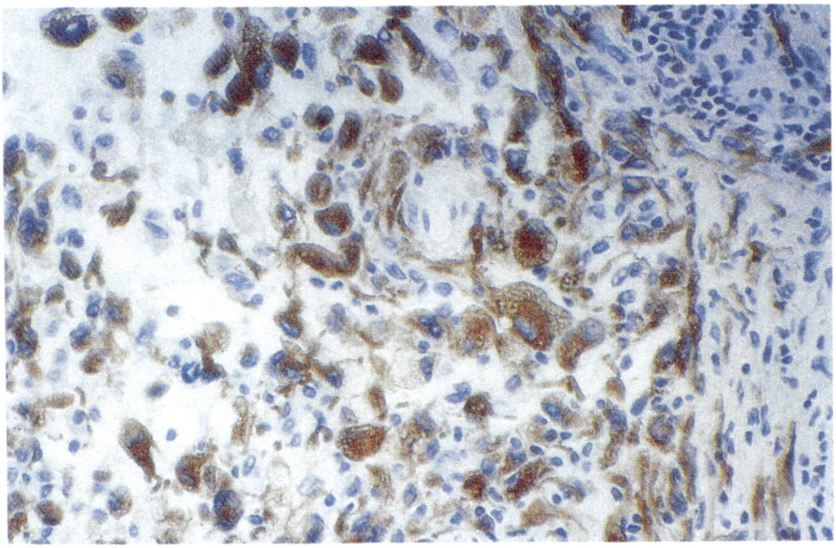

Fig. 18. *Pleomorphic xanthoastrocytoma* with numerous foamy, GFAP expressing cells

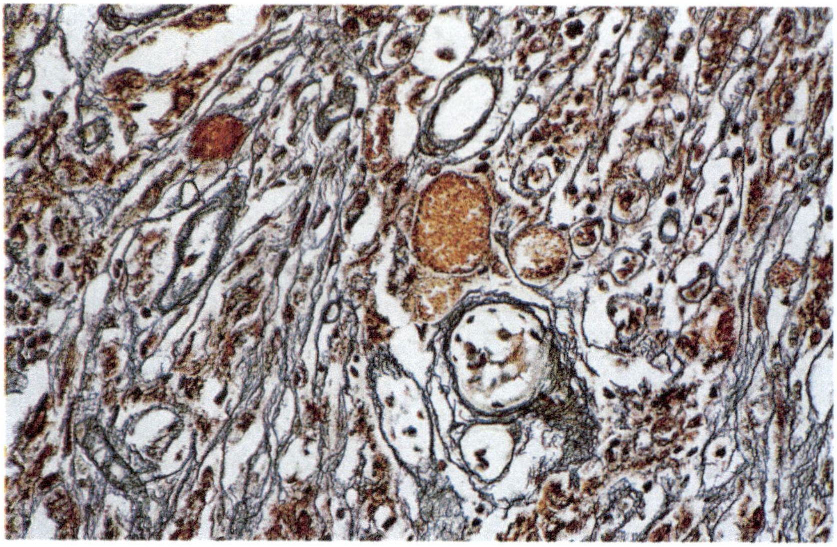

Fig. 19. *Pleomorphic xanthoastrocytoma.* Tumor cells are surrounded by a dense, intercellular reticulin network

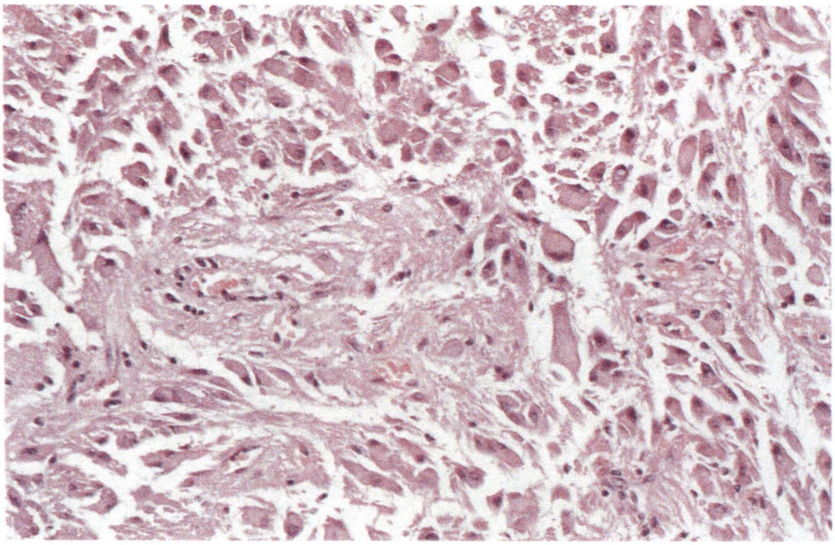

Fig. 20. *Subependymal giant cell astrocytoma* with perivascular arrangement of tumour cells in a patient with tuberous sclerosis

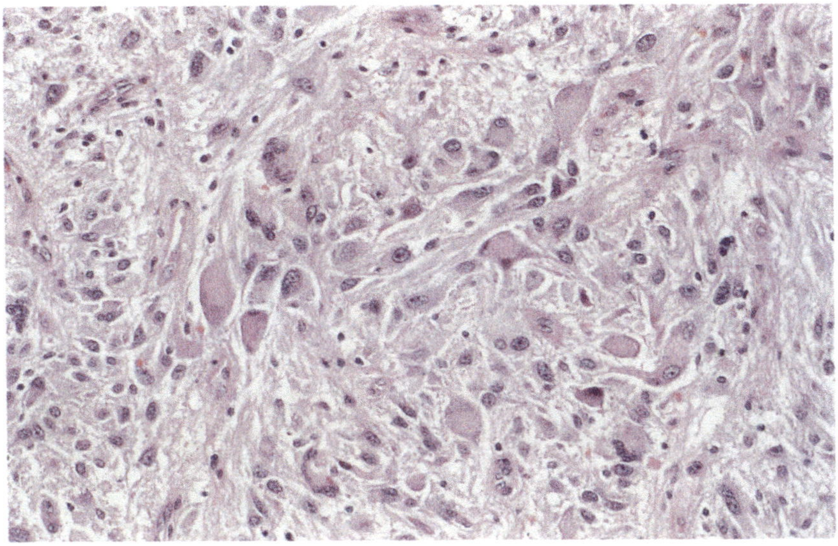

Fig. 21. *Subependymal giant cell astrocytoma.* Note the superficial resemblance of some tumour cells to neurons

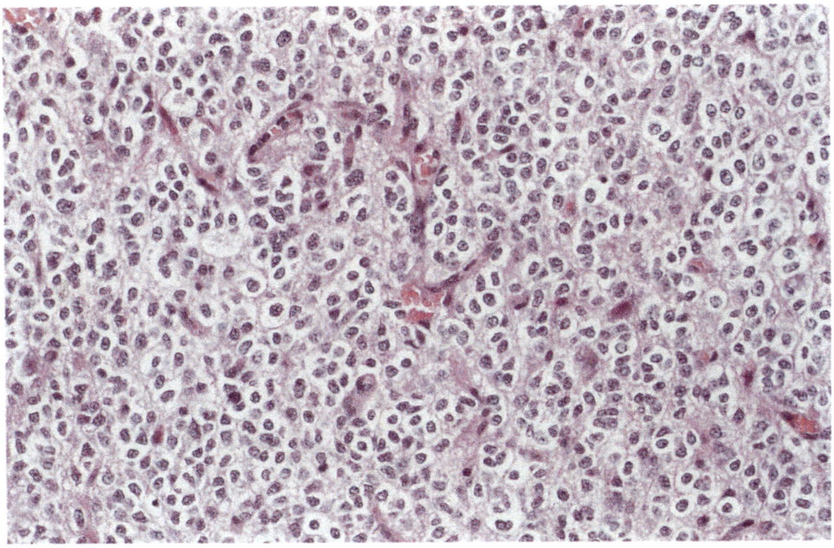

Fig. 22. *Oligodendroglioma.* Nuclei are surrounded by swollen, clear cytoplasm

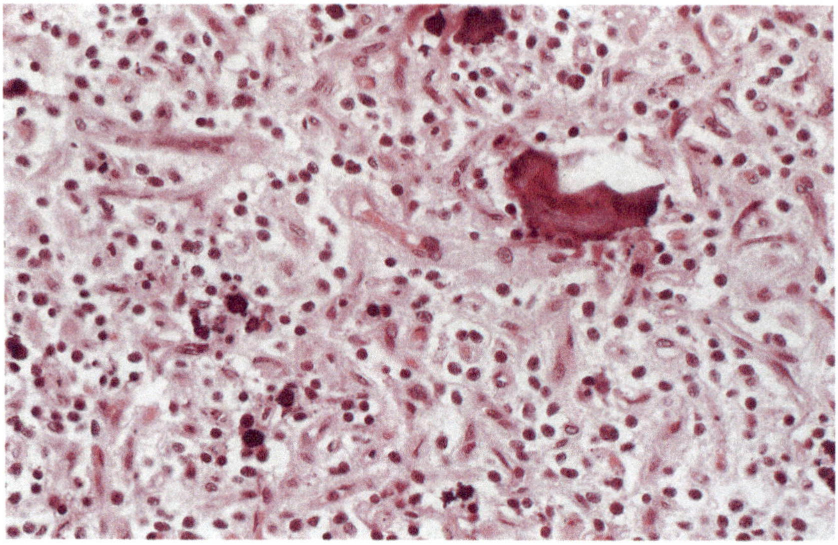

Fig. 23. *Oligodendroglioma* with extensive calcification and delicate, branching vessels

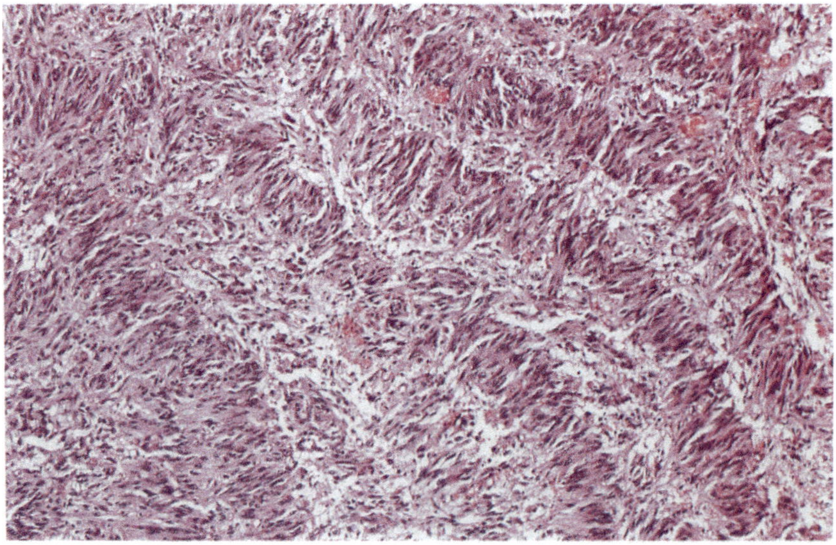

Fig. 24. *Oligodendroglioma*. Elongated tumour cells form parallel rows with nuclear palisading

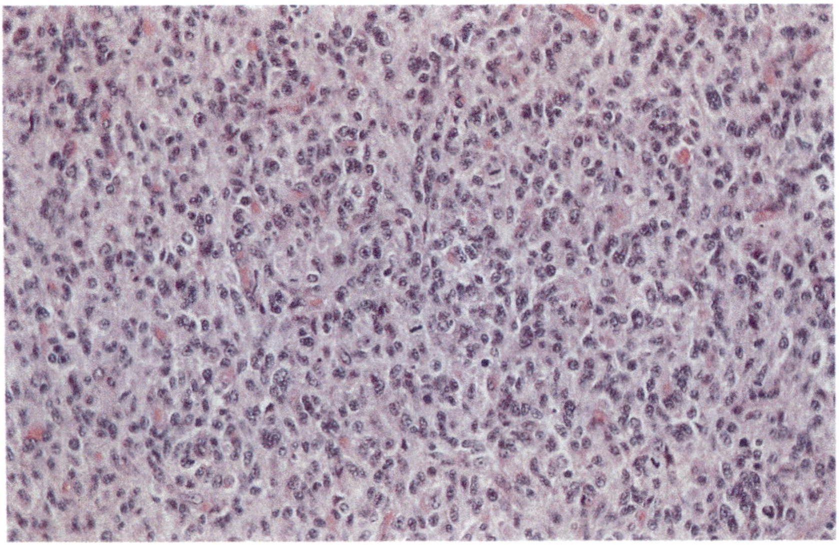

Fig. 25. *Anaplastic oligodendroglioma* with increased cellularity, numerous mitoses and nuclear atypia

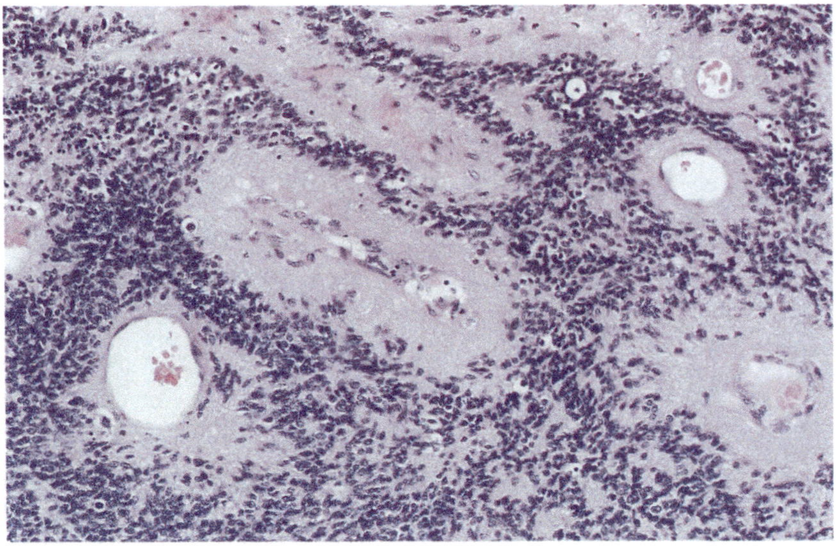

Fig. 26. *Ependymoma* with typical nuclear-free spaces around vessels (perivascular pseudorosettes)

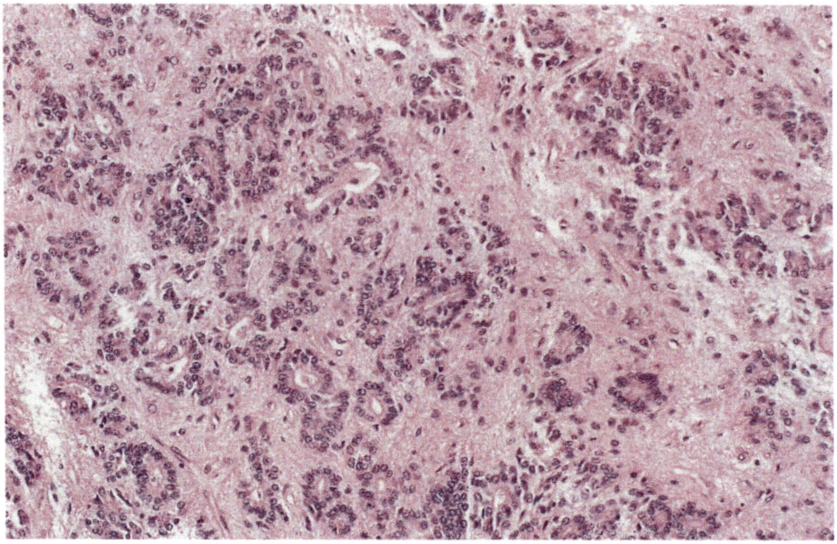

Fig. 27. *Ependymoma*. Numerous ependymal rosettes and tubules

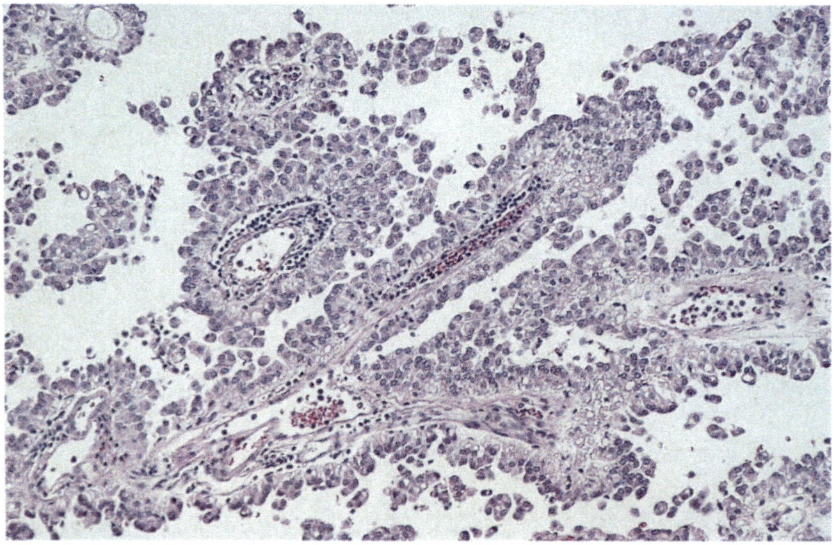

Fig. 28. *Papillary ependymoma*. Tumour cells arranged in a papillary pattern with pseudorosette formation

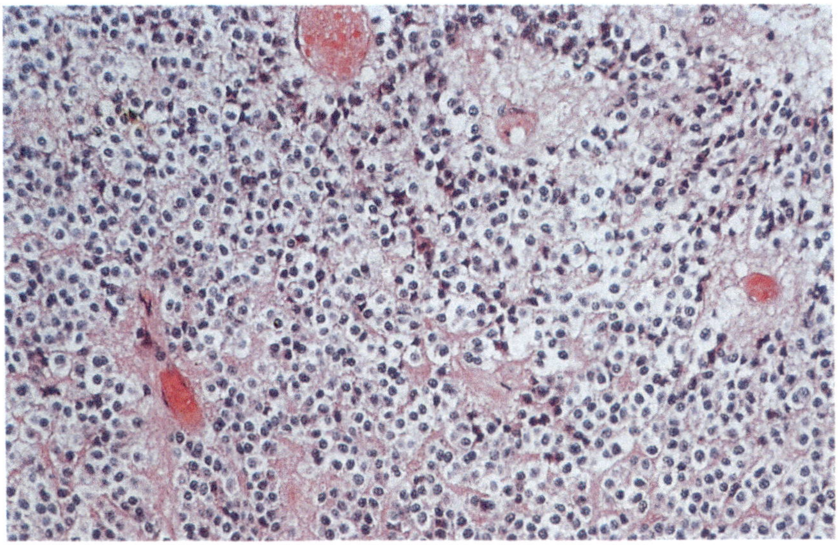

Fig. 29. *Clear cell ependymoma.* Tumour cells have a clear cytoplasm with well defined plasma membrane, superficially resembling neoplastic oligodendrocytes

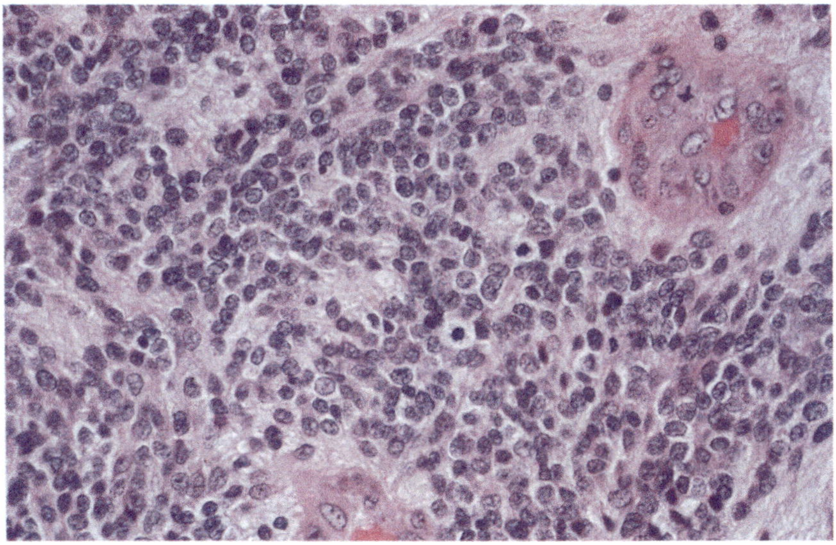

Fig. 30. *Anaplastic ependymoma.* Increased cellularity, numerous mitoses and marked vascular endothelial proliferation

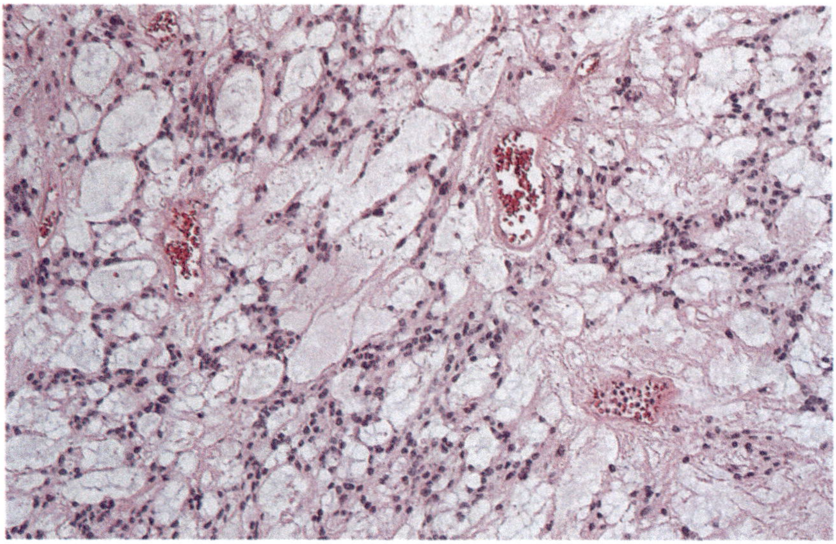

Fig.31. *Myxopapillary ependymoma.* Pools of mucin are surrounded by neoplastic ependymal cells

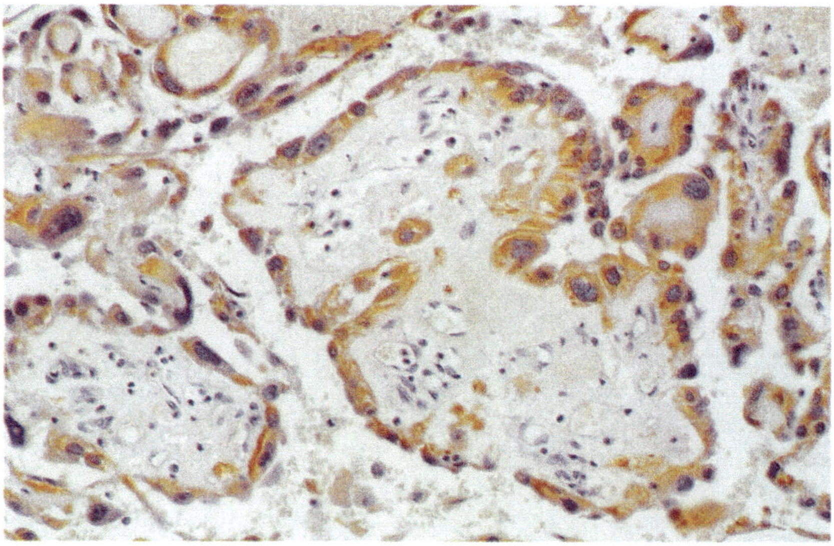

Fig.32. *Myxopapillary ependymoma.* Cuboidal tumour cells surround mucinous or hyalinized vessels and strongly express GFAP

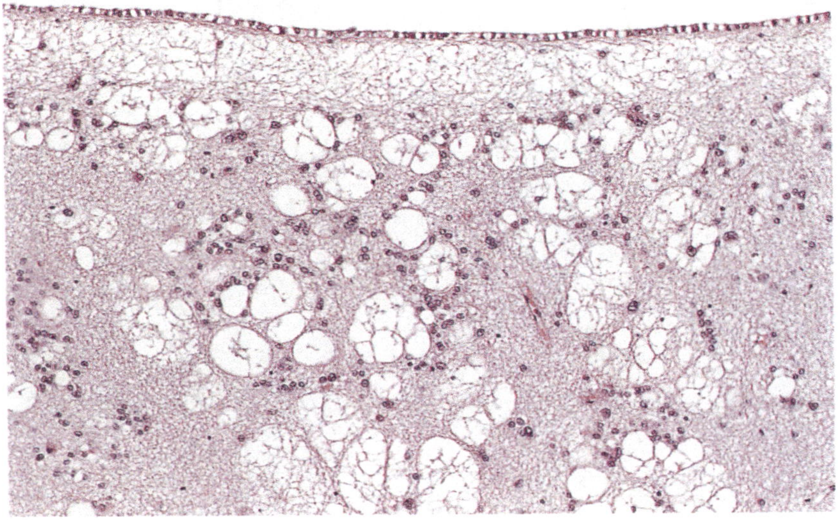

Fig.33. *Subependymoma* of the lateral ventricle with prominent microcyst formation. Note the ependymal lining

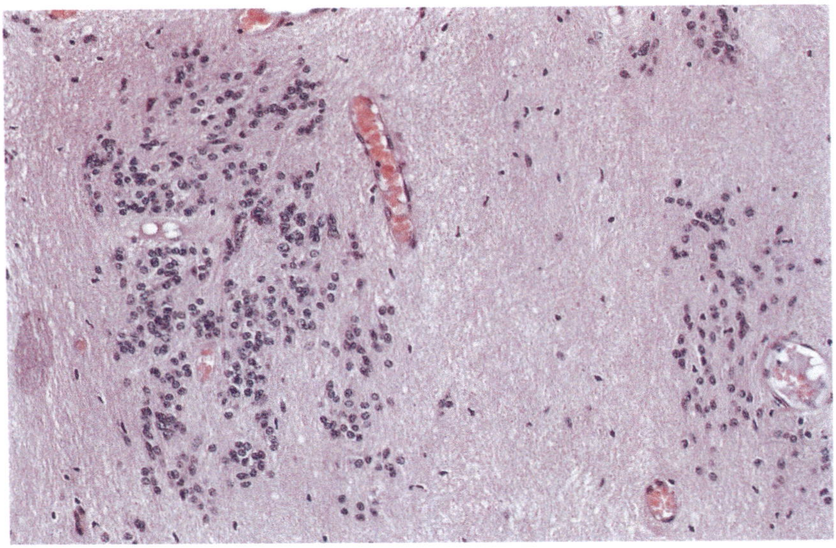

Fig.34. *Subependymoma.* Clusters of tumour cells in a dense fibrillary matrix

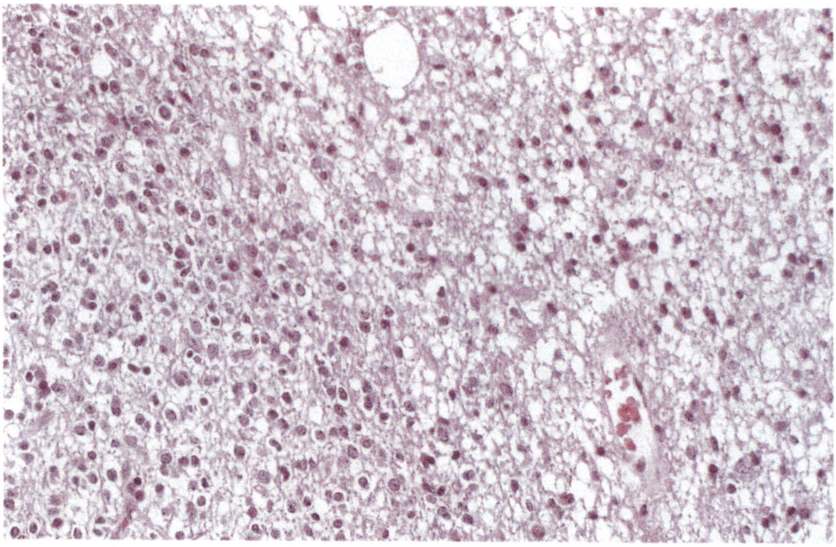

Fig.35. *Oligo-astrocytoma*. Focus of neoplastic oligodendrocytes (left) next to a less cellular area with astrocytic differentiation

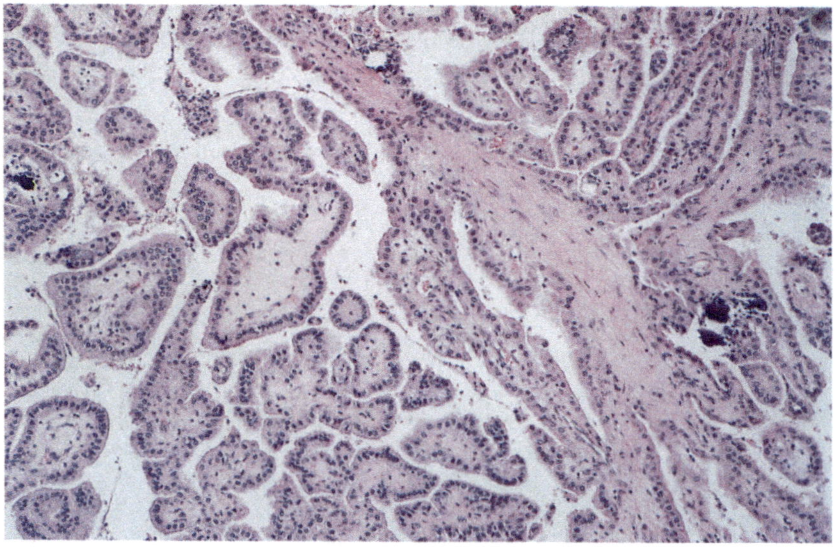

Fig.36. *Choroid plexus papilloma*. Highly differentiated cuboidal cells cover papillary connective tissue cores. Occasional calcifications are typical

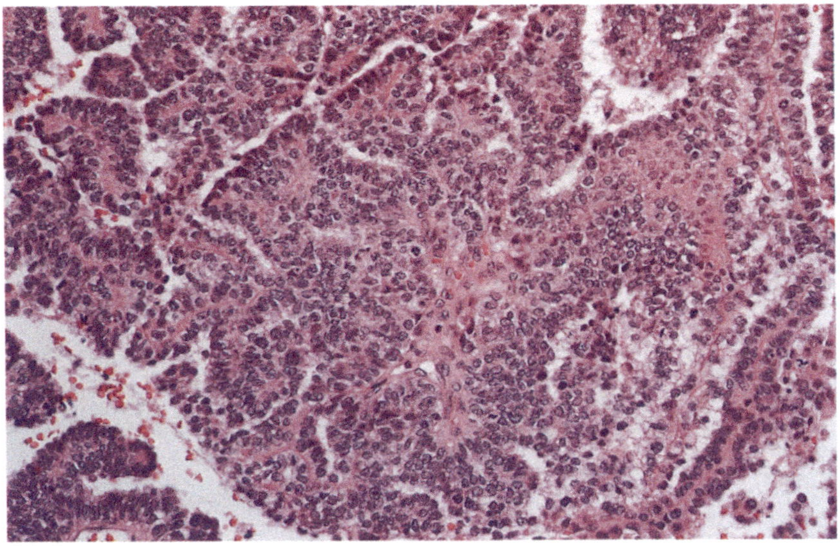

Fig.37. *Choroid plexus carcinoma.* Anaplastic, often multilayered tumour cells with frequent mitoses

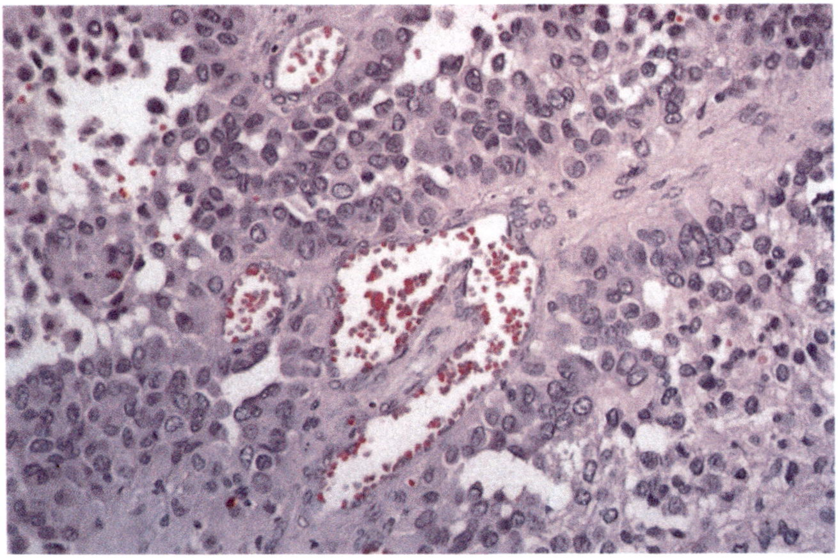

Fig.38. *Astroblastoma.* GFAP expressing neoplastic astrocytes with broad processes radiating towards central blood vessels

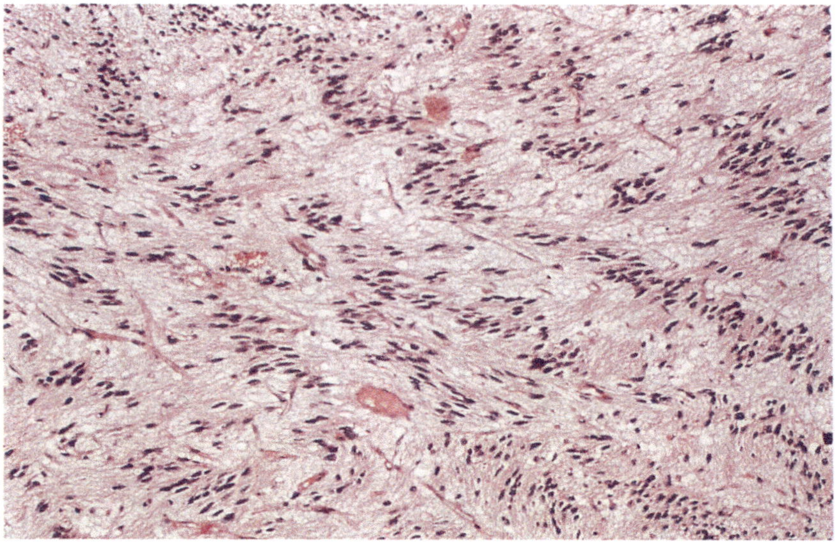

Fig. 39. *Polar spongioblastoma.* Bipolar tumour cells form a typical palisading pattern

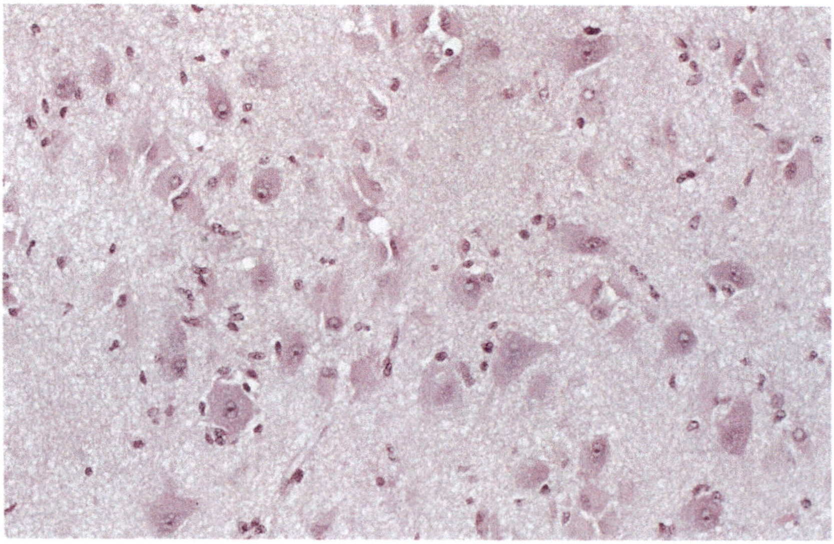

Fig. 40. *Gangliocytoma.* Dysplastic, mature, occasionally binucleate ganglion cells and inconspicuous non-neoplastic glial cells

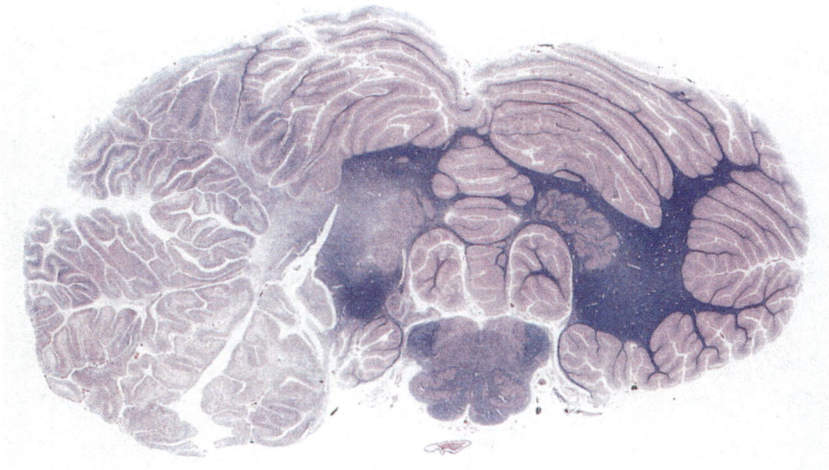

Fig.41. *Dysplastic gangliocytoma of the cerebellum (Lhermitte-Duclos)* with marked enlargement of the folia of the affected left cerebellar hemisphere

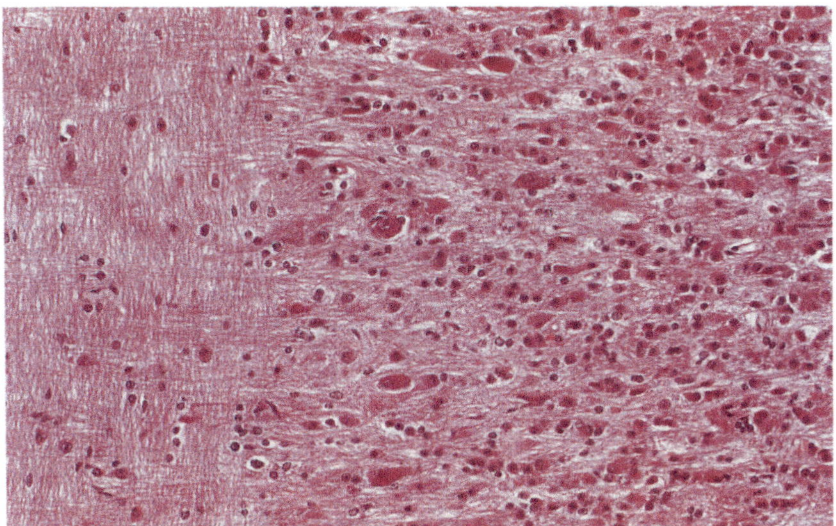

Fig.42. *Dysplastic gangliocytoma of the cerebellum (Lhermitte-Duclos).* Accumulation of dysplastic granular cells which often resemble Purkinje neurons

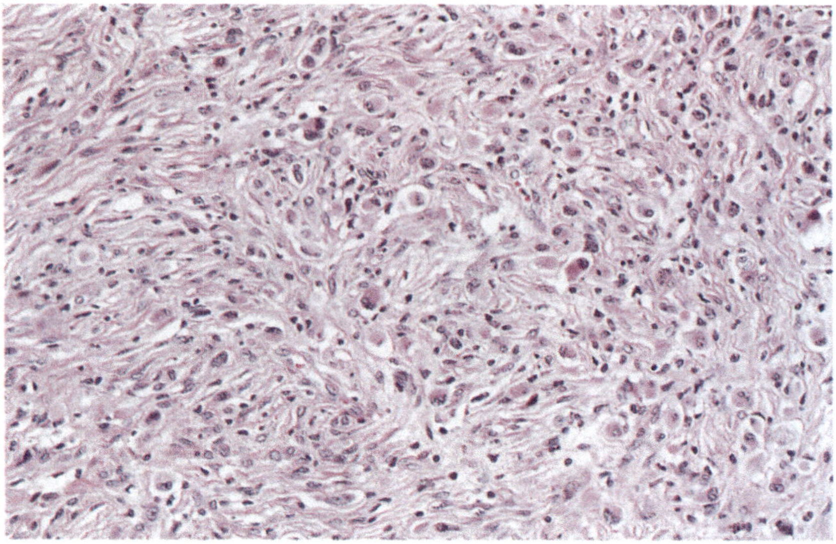

Fig.43. *Desmoplastic infantile ganglioglioma.* Mixed glial-neuronal neoplasm with a marked desmoplastic component

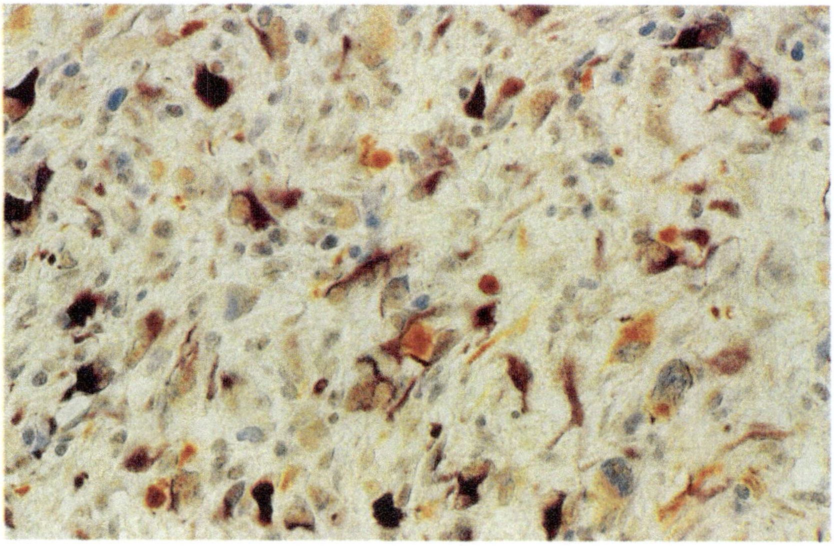

Fig.44. *Desmoplastic infantile ganglioglioma.* Double immunohistochemical staining showing neuronal (neurofilament protein, brown) and glial (GFAP, purple/blue) differentiation

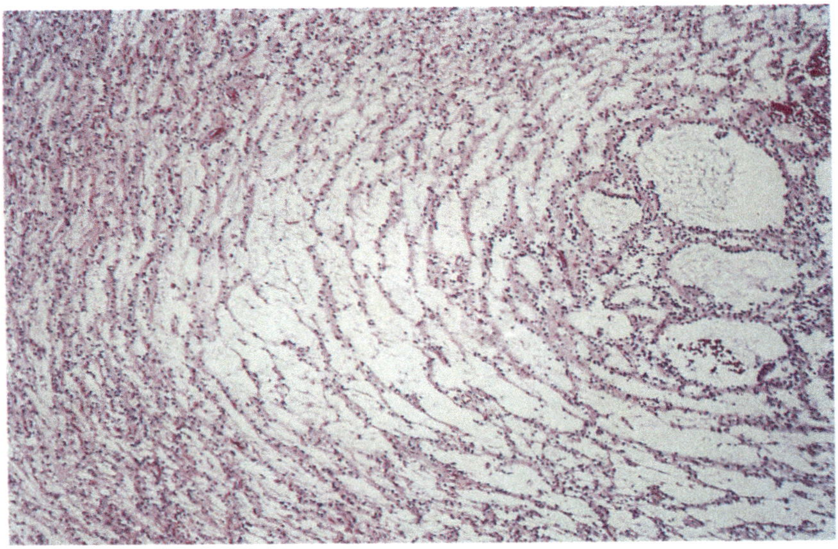

Fig. 45. *Dysembryoplastic neuroepithelial tumour (DNT).* Oligodendroglial tumour cells form a cortical nodule with a loosely textured, target-like pattern

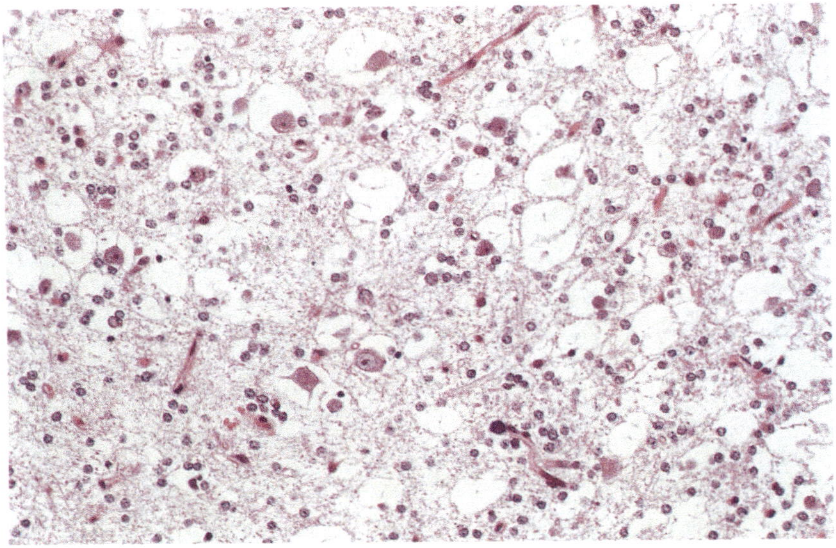

Fig. 46. *Dysembryoplastic neuroepithelial tumour (DNT).* Neurons appear to float in spaces within a glial matrix containing predominantly oligodendrocytes

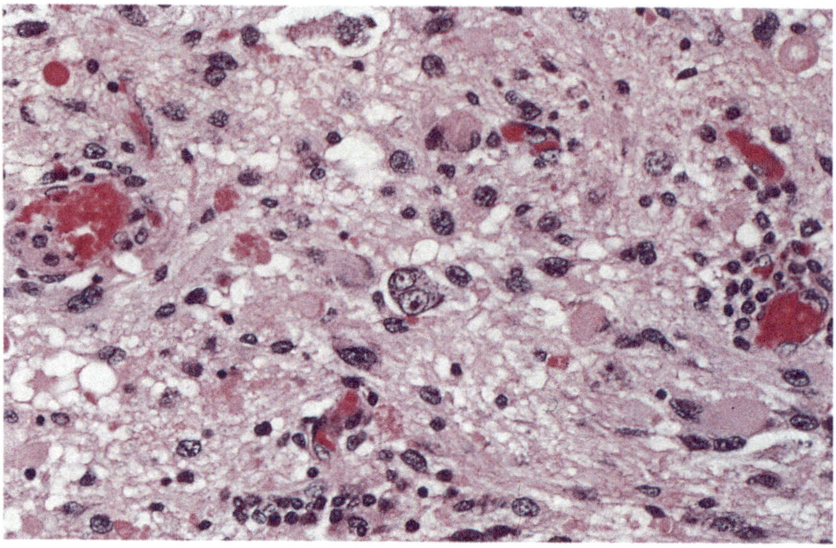

Fig. 47. *Ganglioglioma.* Mixed glial-neuronal neoplasm with occasionally binucleate ganglion cells (center) and perivascular lymphocytic infiltrates

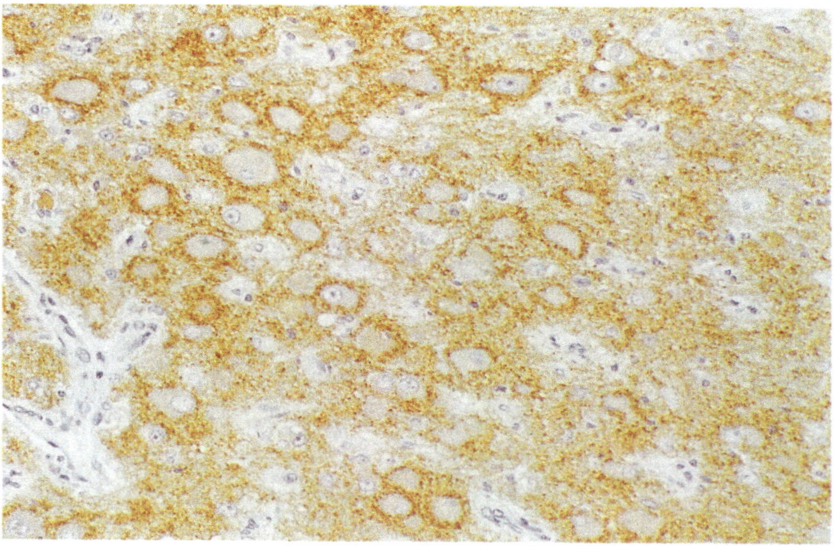

Fig. 48. *Ganglioglioma.* Immunoreactivity for synaptophysin is accentuated at synapses along the neuronal plasma membrane

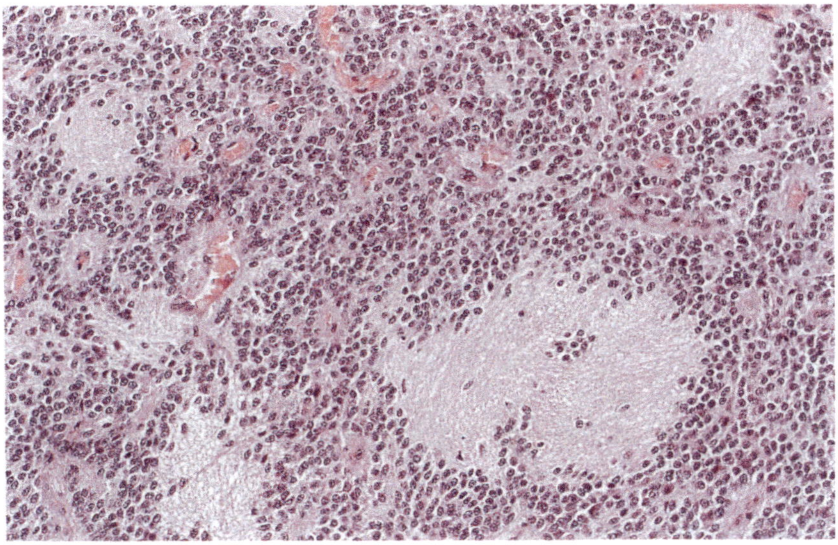

Fig. 49. *Central neurocytoma.* Isomorphic round tumour cell nuclei with occasional nuclear-free neuropil islands

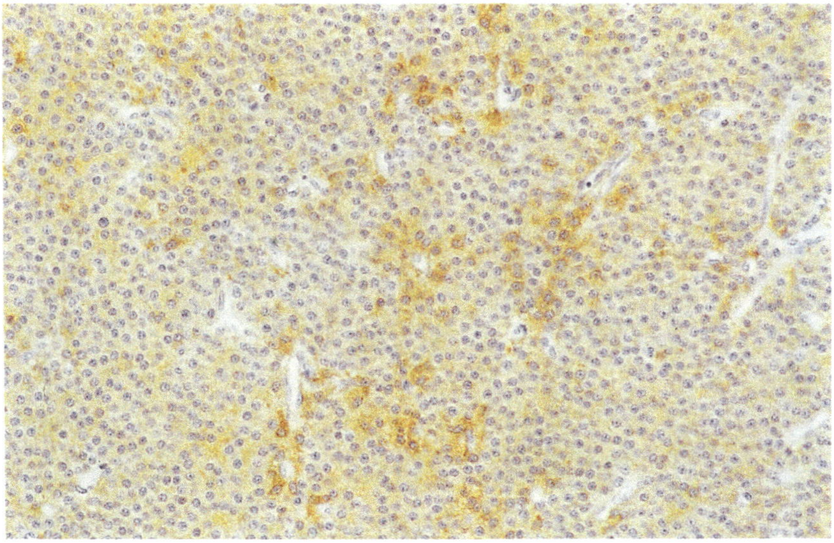

Fig. 50. *Central neurocytoma.* Consistent, though variable expression of the neuronal marker protein, synaptophysin

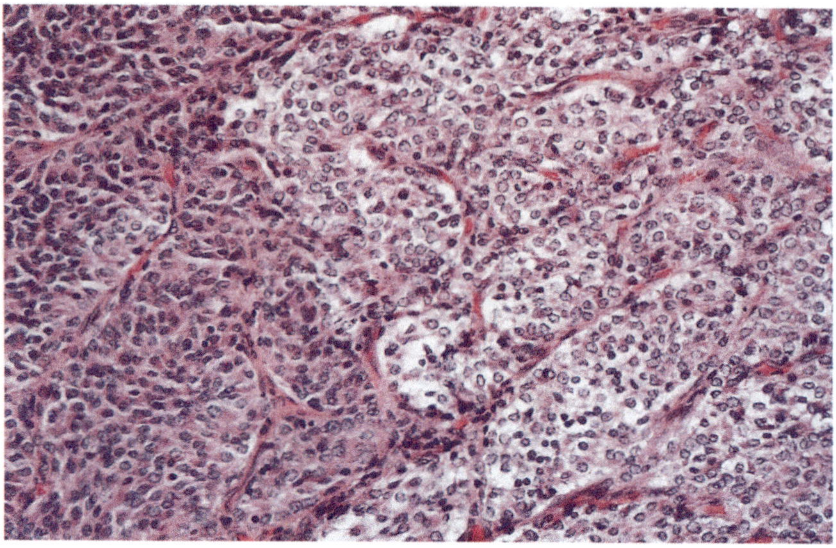

Fig. 51. *Olfactory neuroblastoma.* Nodules of neoplastic neuroblasts in a vascularized stroma

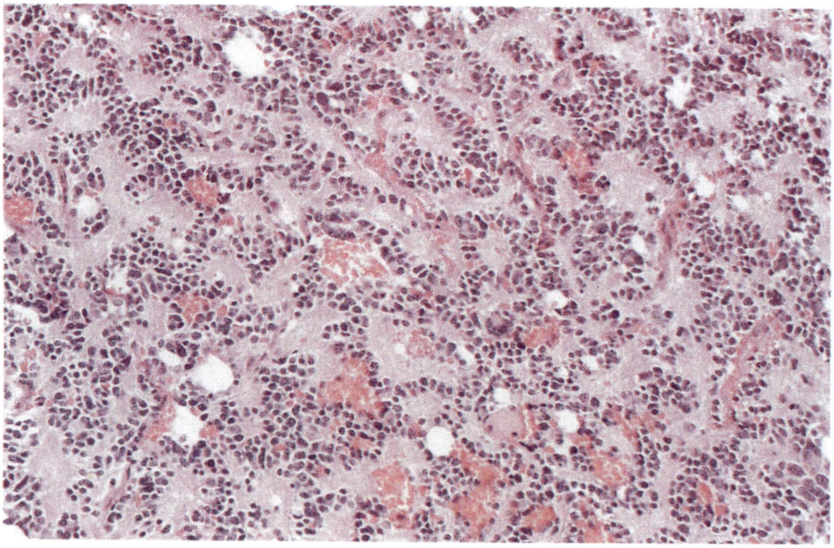

Fig. 52. *Pineocytoma.* Neoplastic pineal parenchymal cells forming large rosettes

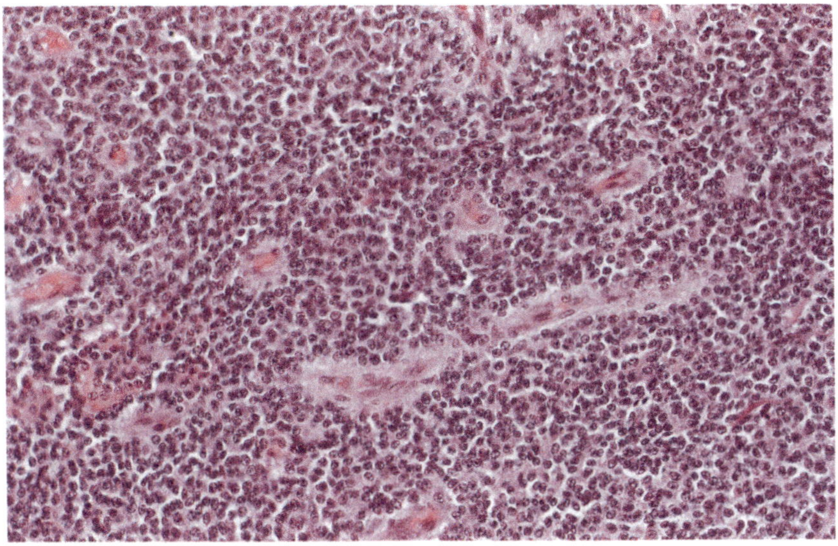

Fig. 53. *Pineoblastoma.* Immature, highly cellular embryonal tumour without detectable pineocytic differentiation

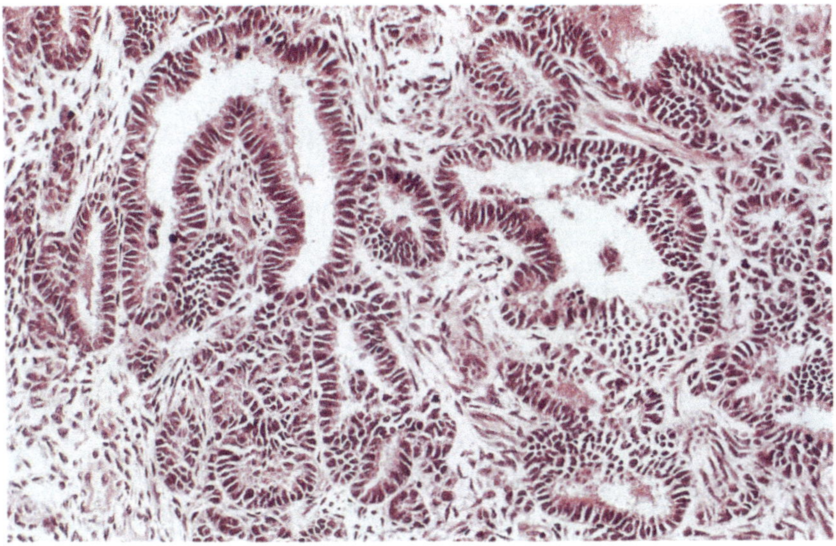

Fig. 54. *Medulloepithelioma.* Primitive neuroectodermal cells resting on a basement membrane form typical glandular structures

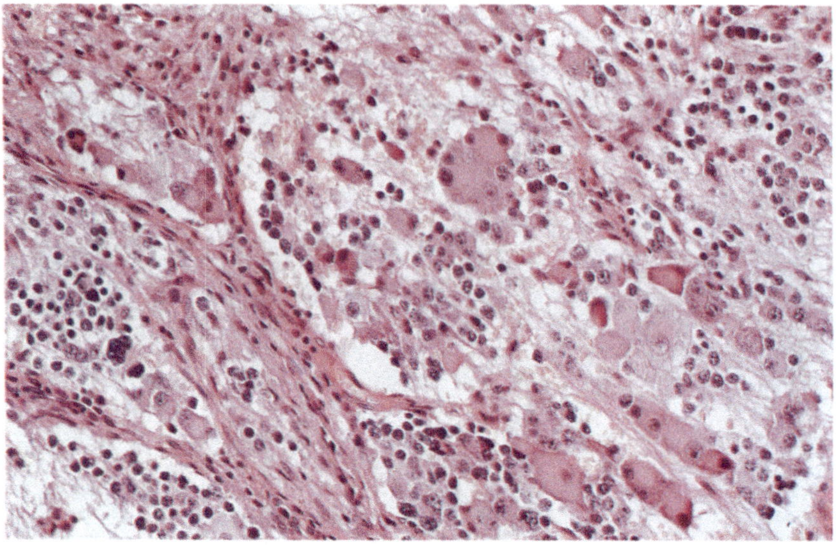

Fig. 55. *Ganglioneuroblastoma.* Small, neoplastic neuroblasts and foci of advanced neuronal differentiation with mature, often multinucleate ganglion cells

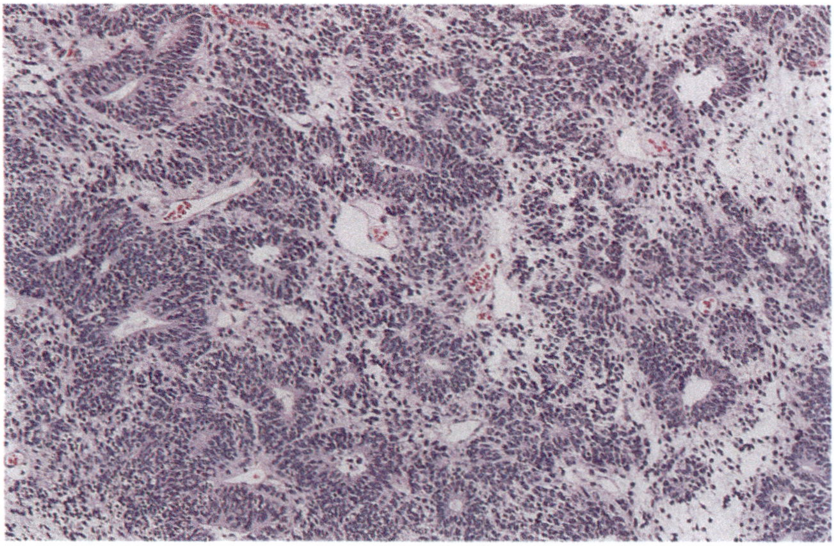

Fig. 56. *Ependymoblastoma.* Highly cellular embryonal tumour with numerous ependymoblastic, multi-layered rosettes with a lumen

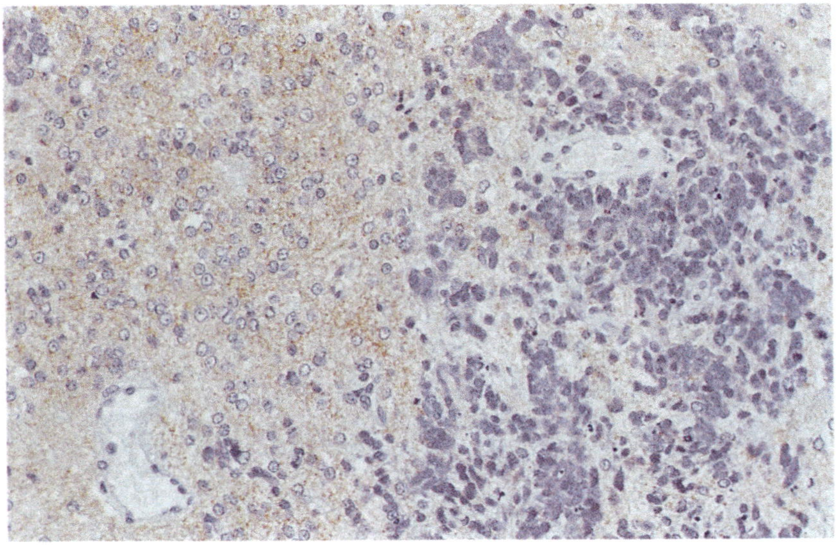

Fig.57. *Primitive neuroectodermal tumour (PNET)* located in the parietal lobe of a two year-old child. The tumor area on the left shows incipient neuronal differentiation with synaptophysin expression

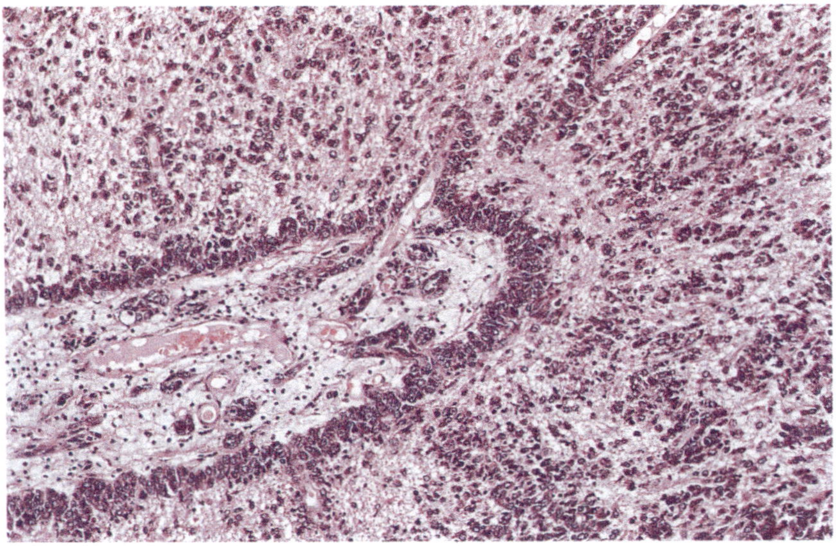

Fig.58. *Medulloblastoma.* Extensive infiltration of the subpial region and of the molecular layer of the cerebellum. Clusters of tumour cells are also observed in the subarachnoidal space

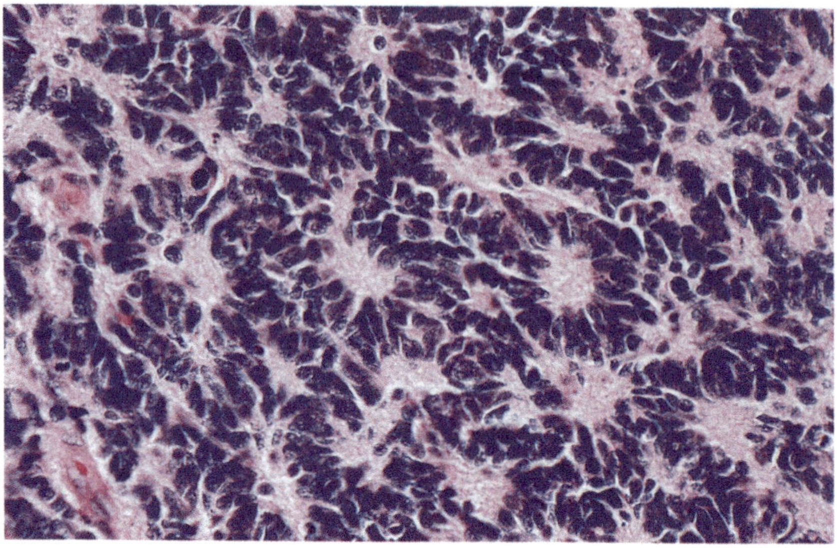

Fig.59. *Medulloblastoma.* Primitive, undifferentiated tumour cells with carrot-shaped nuclei and numerous neuroblastic (Homer Wright) rosettes

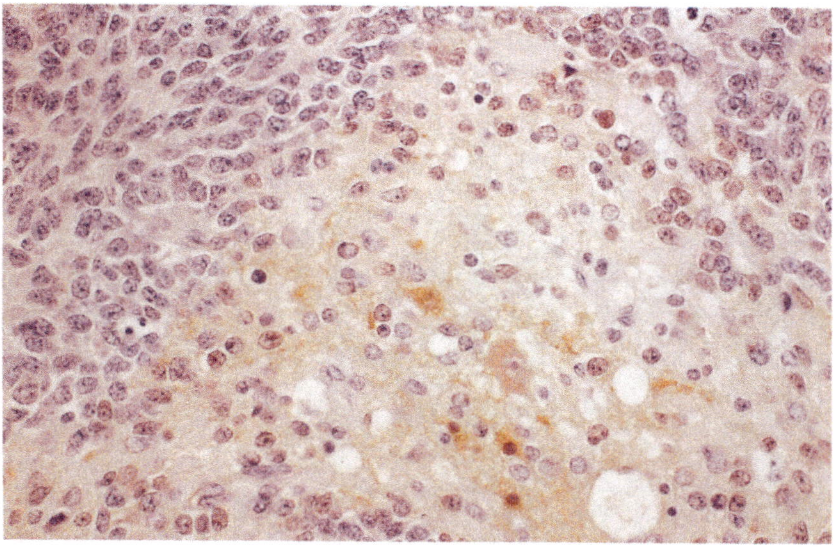

Fig.60. *Medulloblastoma.* Focal neuronal differentiation with mature ganglion cells and expression of neuron-specific enolase (NSE)

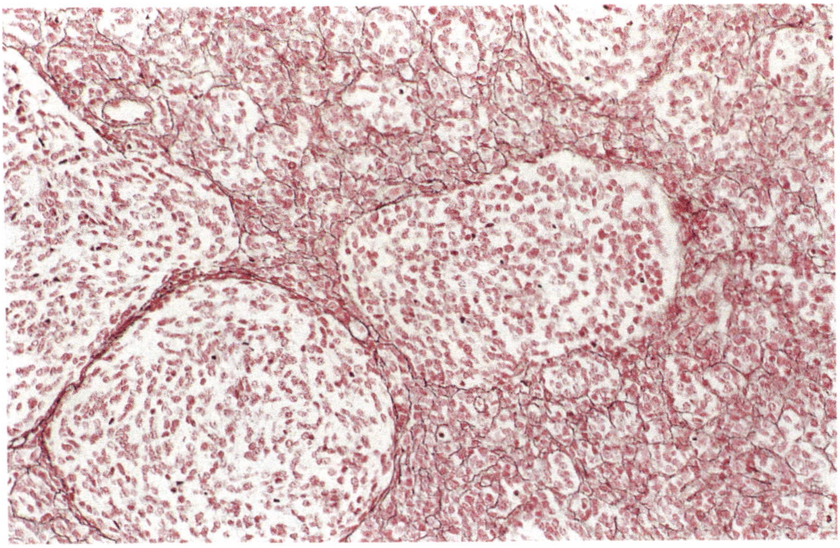

Fig.61. *Desmoplastic medulloblastoma.* Tumour cells form a dense intercellular reticulin network with pale, reticulin-free islands

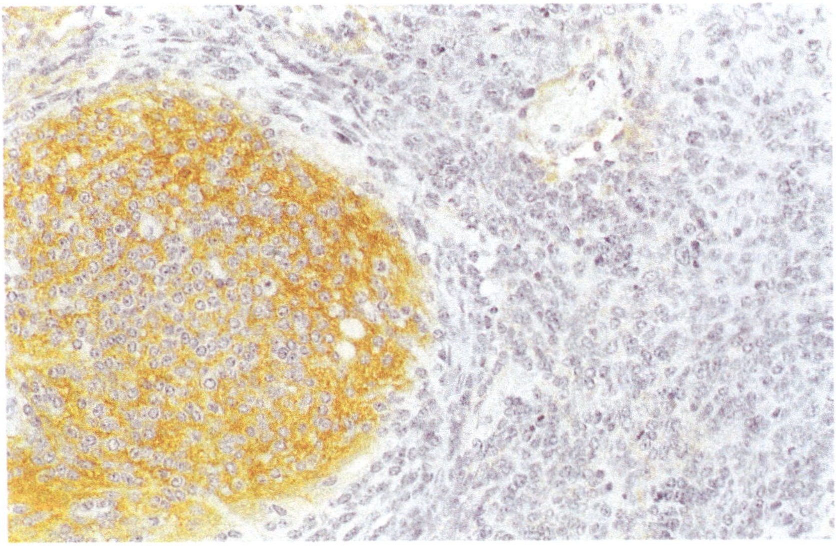

Fig.62. *Desmoplastic medulloblastoma.* Reticulin-free island with marked expression of the neuronal marker protein, synaptophysin

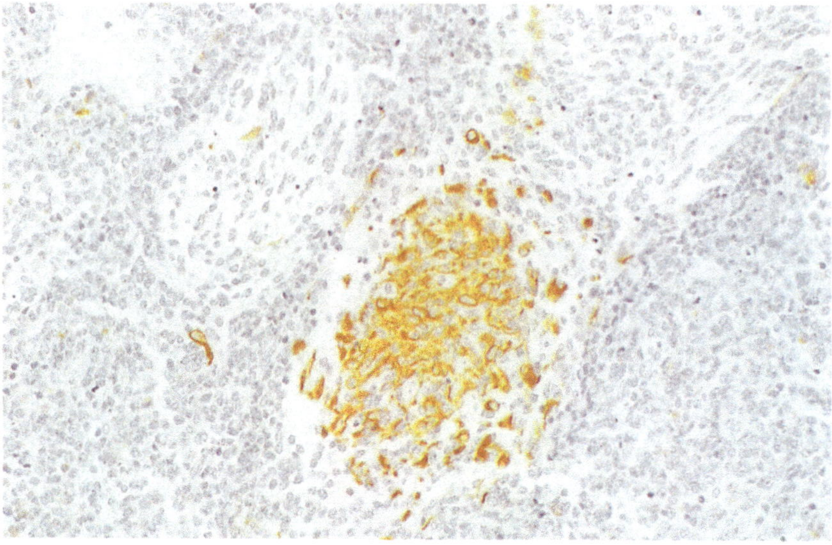

Fig. 63. *Desmoplastic medulloblastoma.* Astrocytic differentiation with GFAP expression is restricted to the reticulin-free islands

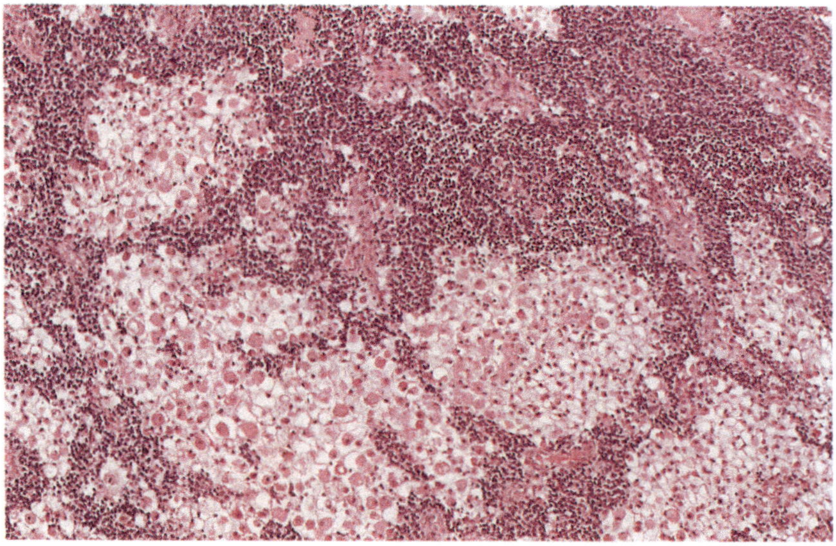

Fig. 64. *Medullomyoblastoma.* Primitive medulloblastoma cells alternate with foci containing large, eosinophilic neoplastic myocytes

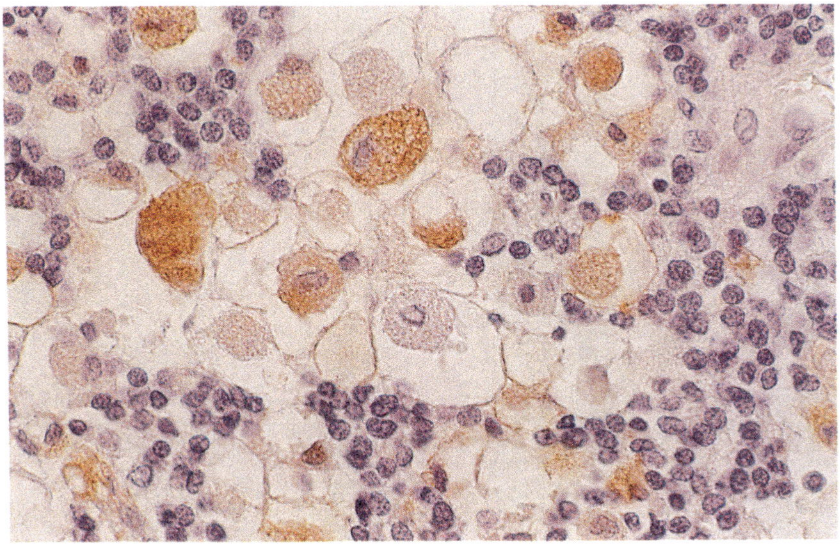

Fig. 65. *Medullomyoblastoma.* Tumour cells with myoblastic differentiation and variable immunoreactivity for myoglobin

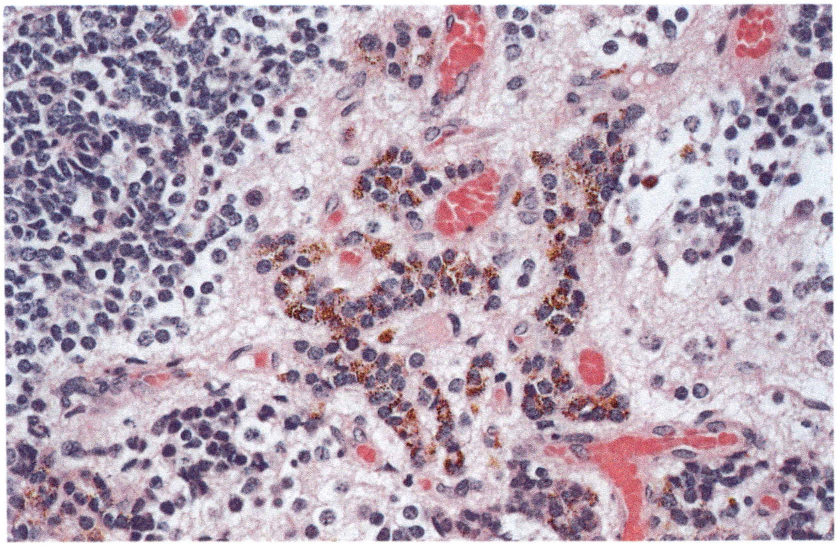

Fig. 66. *Melanotic medulloblastoma.* Foci of epithelial, melanin-containing tumour cells

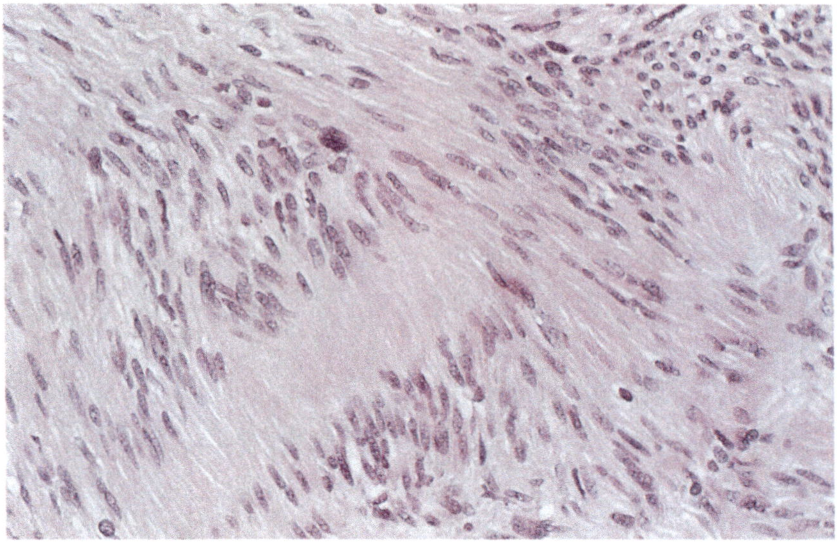

Fig. 67. *Schwannoma.* Neoplastic Schwann cells organized in a typical palisading pattern

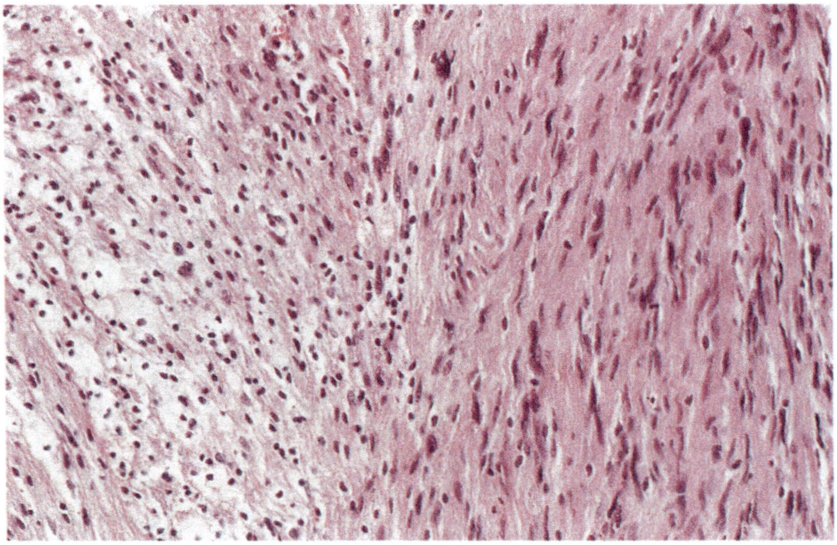

Fig. 68. *Schwannoma* of the acoustic nerve. Areas with compact elongated neoplastic Schwann cells (Antoni A) alternate with a less cellular pattern characterized by marked lipidization (Antoni B)

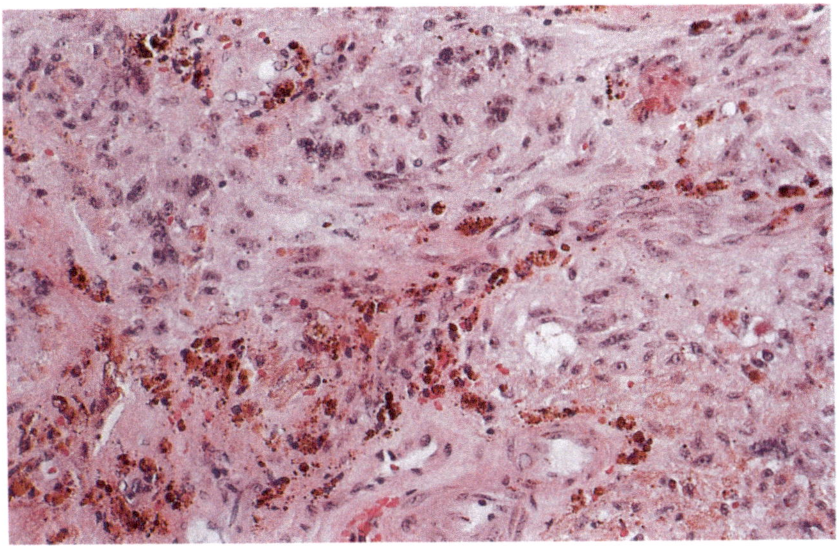

Fig. 69. *Melanotic schwannoma.* Numerous tumour cells contain melanin

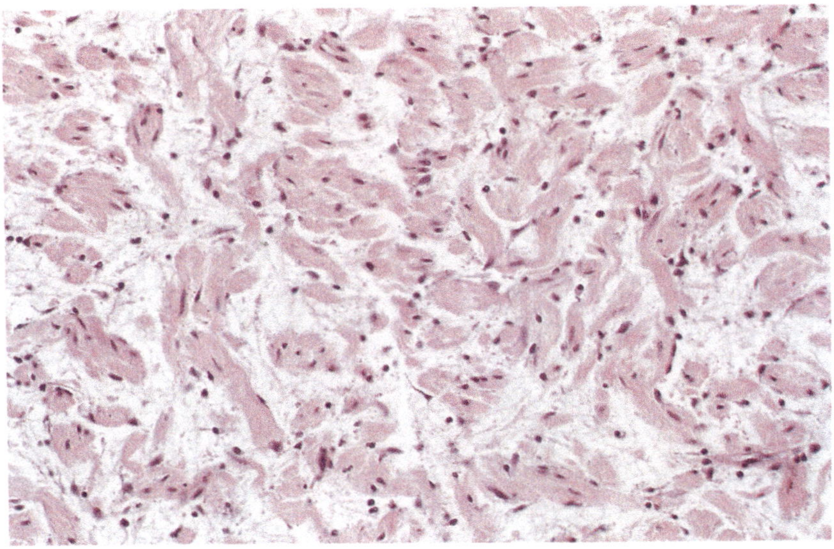

Fig. 70. *Neurofibroma.* Wavy, elongated tumour cells in a loose, myxoid matrix

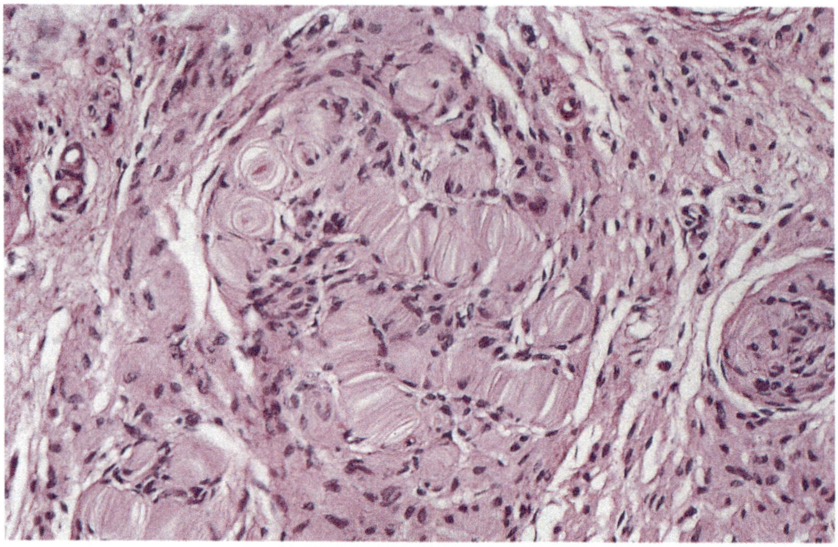

Fig.71. *Neurofibroma* with focal palisading (Meissner corpuscules) in a patient with von Recklinghausen disease (neurofibromatosis I)

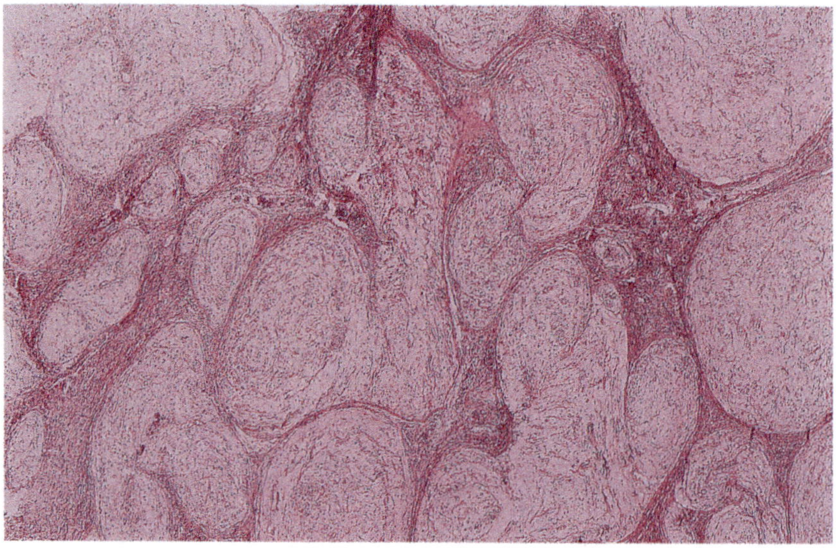

Fig.72. *Plexiform neurofibroma*. Tumour nodules are arranged in racemose pattern and separated by connective tissue

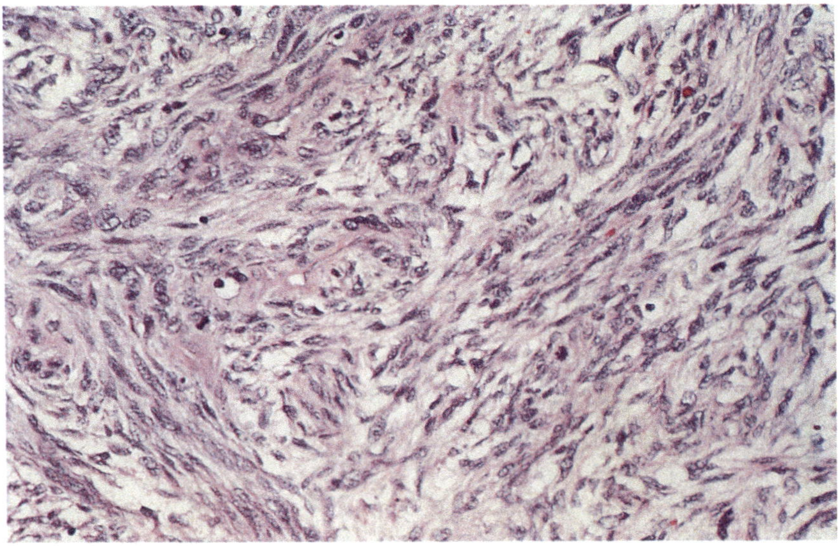

Fig.73. *Malignant peripheral nerve sheath tumour (MPNST).* Highly mitotic, anaplastic tumour cells form an abortive schwannoma-like pattern

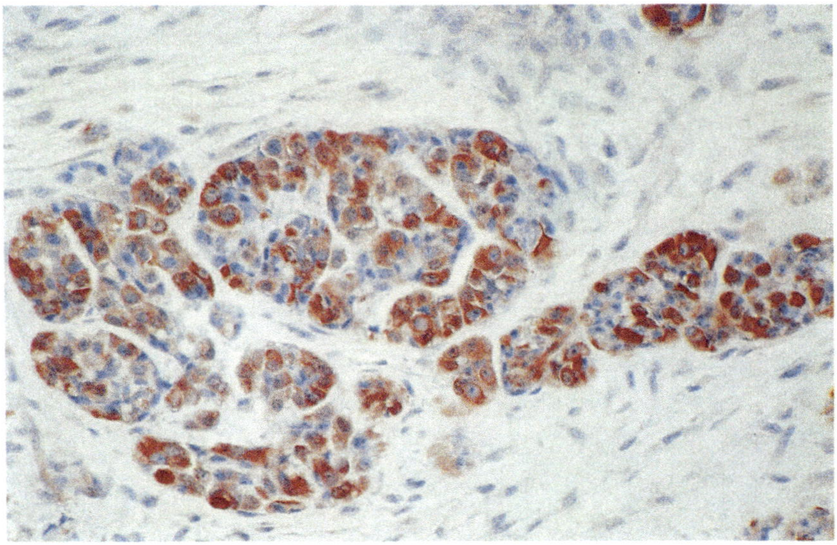

Fig.74. *Epithelioid malignant peripheral nerve sheath tumour (MPNST).* Some tumour cell areas show an epithelioid pattern. Immunoperoxidase for S-100 protein

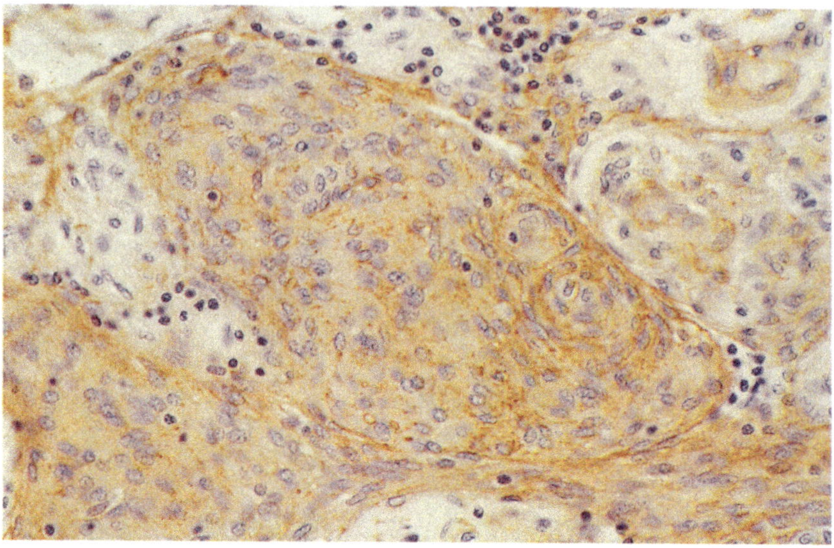

Fig. 75. *Meningothelial meningioma.* Solid lobules of meningothelial cells with ill-defined cell membranes and marked expression of epithelial membrane antigen (EMA)

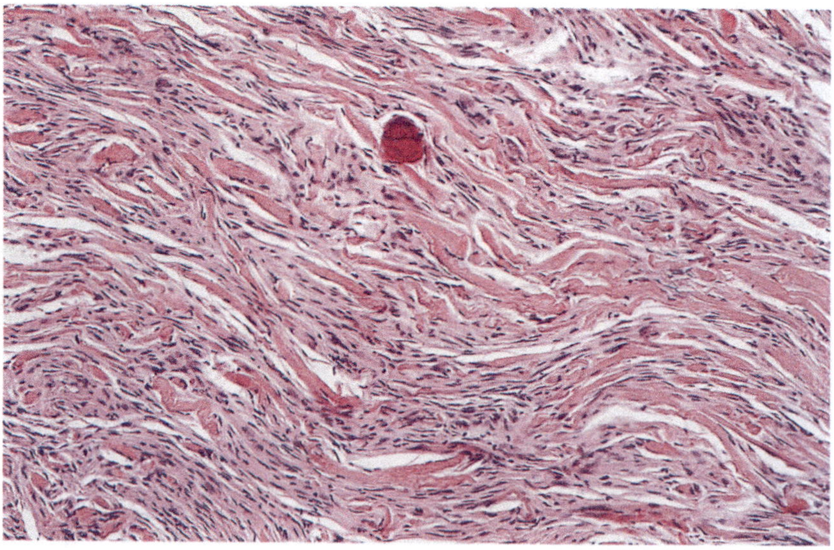

Fig. 76. *Fibrous meningioma.* Parallel and interlacing bundles of fibroblast-like tumour cells with extensive collagen deposition

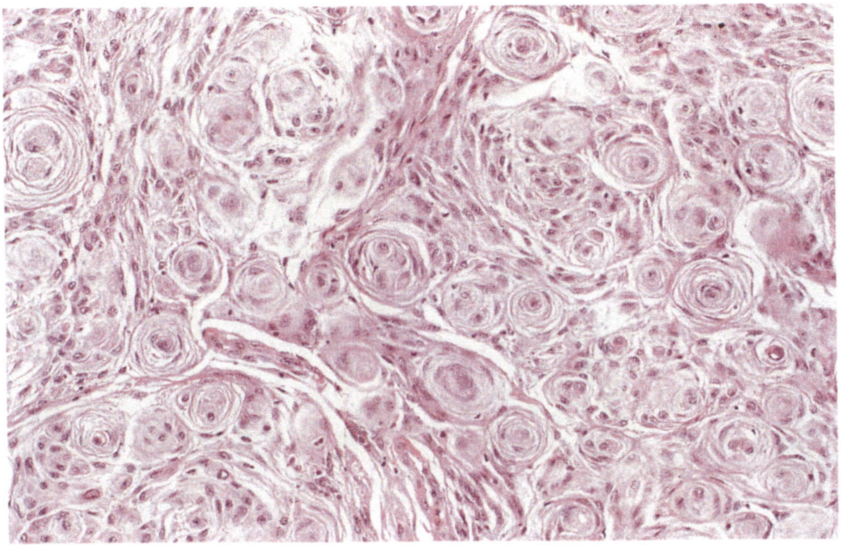

Fig. 77. *Transitional meningioma.* Extensive whorl formation in a meningioma with meningothelial and fibrous features

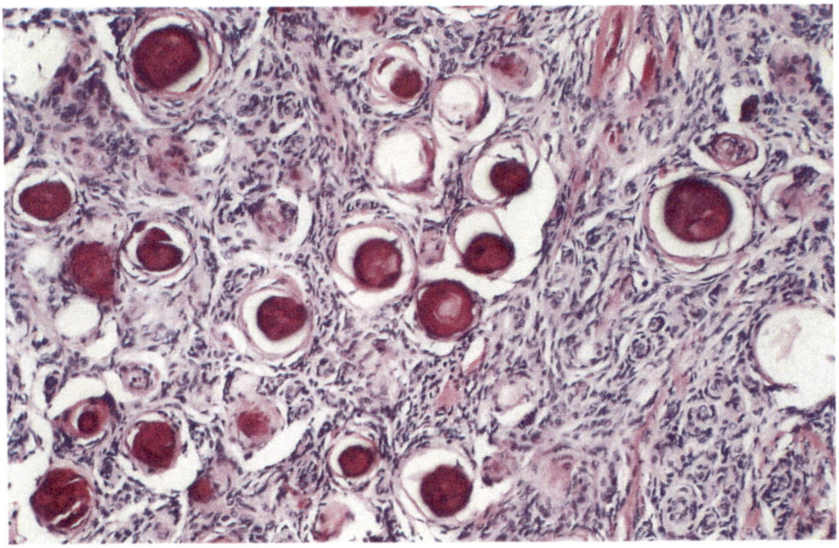

Fig. 78. *Psammomatous meningioma.* Meningioma of the transitional type with abundant, often calcified psammoma bodies

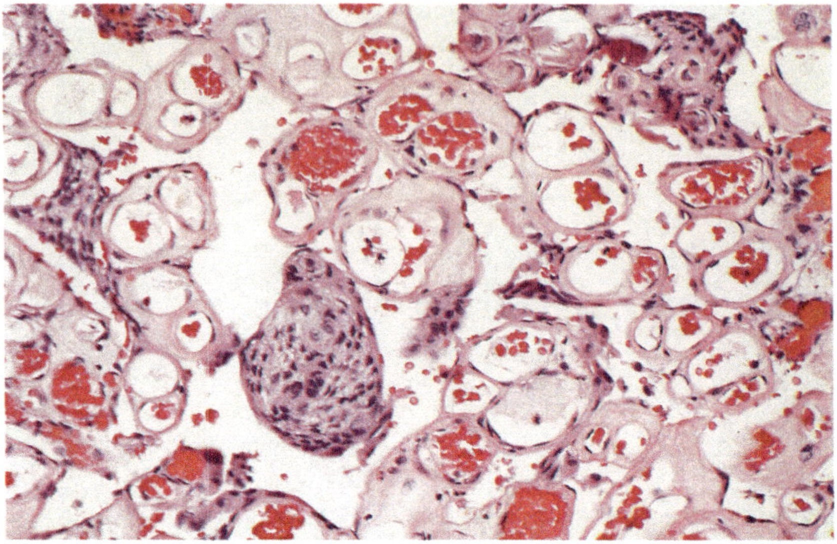

Fig. 79. *Angiomatous meningioma.* Hypervascularized stroma with occasional nests of neoplastic meningothelial cells

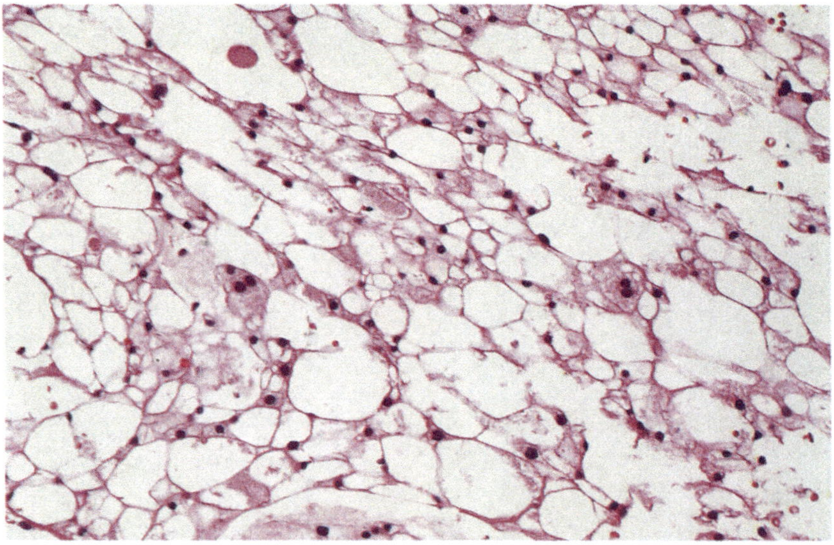

Fig. 80. *Microcystic meningioma.* The histological pattern is characterized by numerous large, intracellular cysts

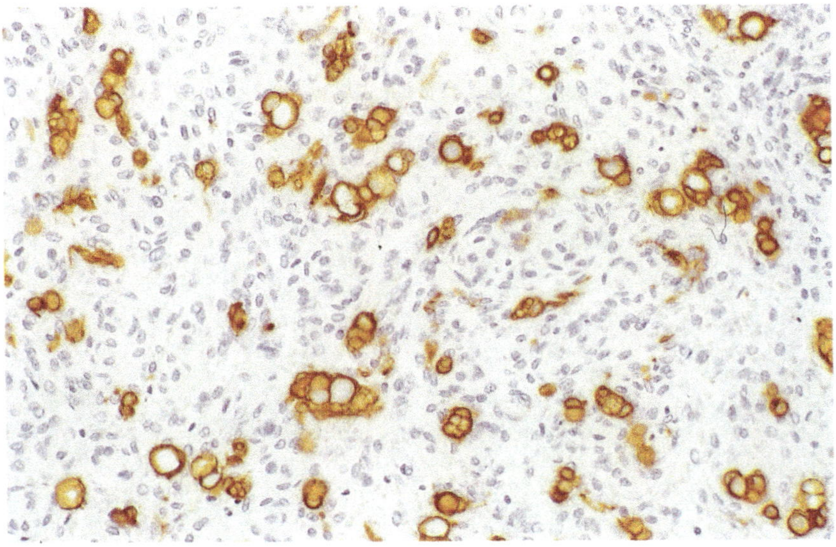

Fig. 81. *Secretory meningioma.* Focal epithelial differentiation with marked immunoreactivity for cytokeratin

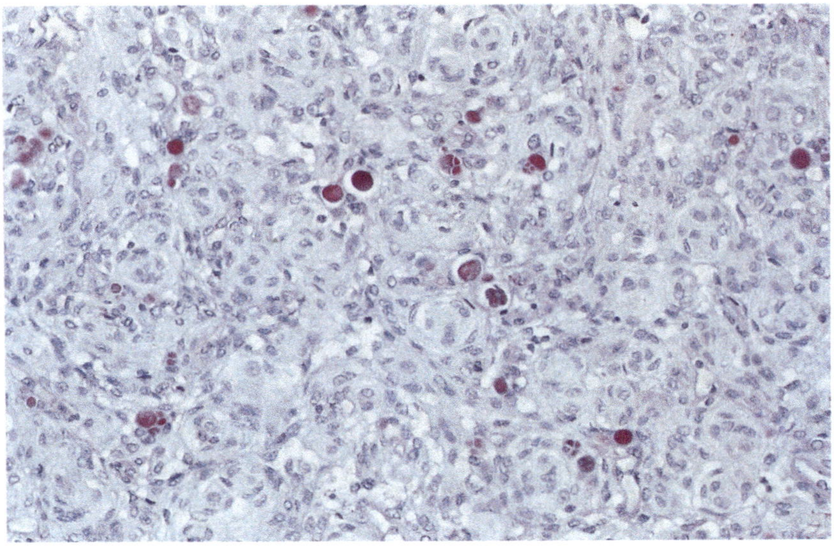

Fig. 82. *Secretory meningioma.* Glandular lumina often contain PAS-positive globules

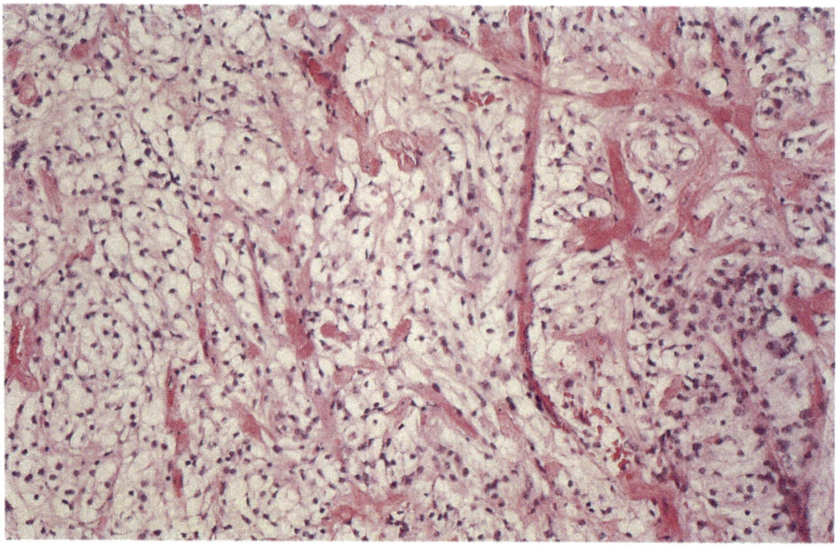

Fig.83. *Clear cell meningioma.* Patternless meningioma with polygonal, clear tumour cells rich in glycogen

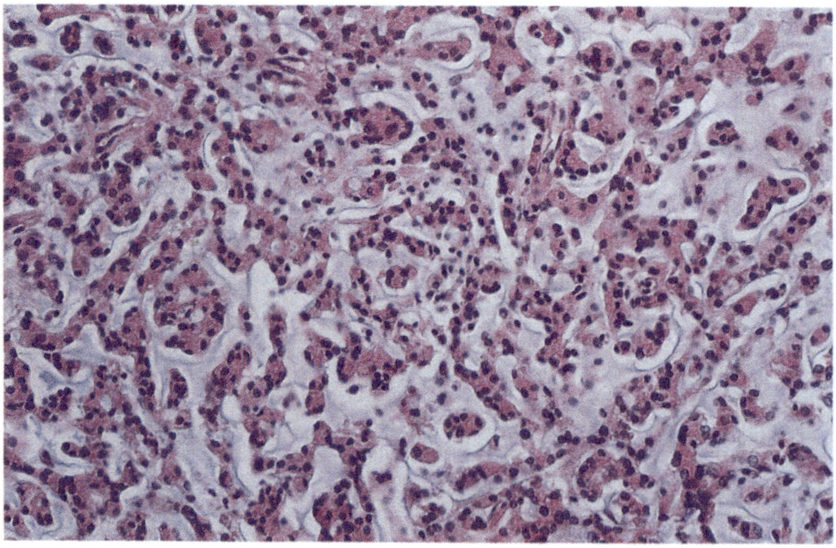

Fig.84. *Chordoid meningioma.* Chordoma-like chains of eosinophilic tumour cells in a mucous-rich matrix

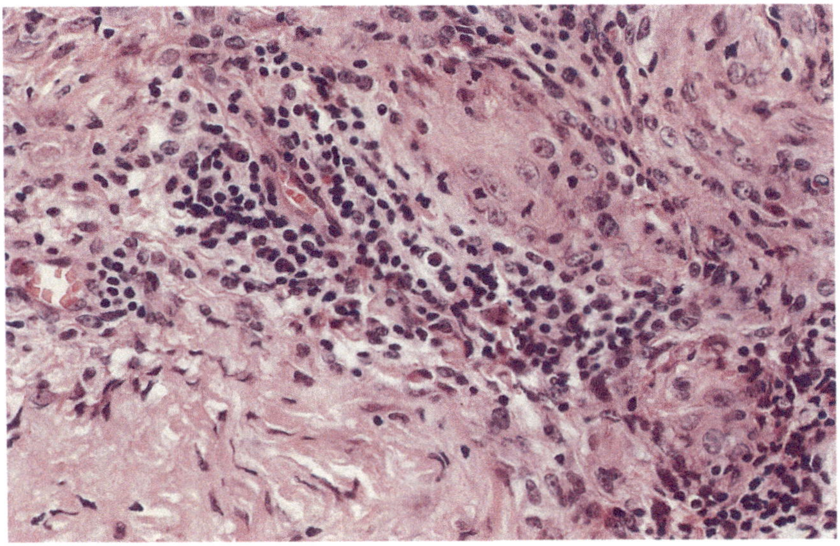

Fig.85. *Lymphoplasmacyte-rich meningioma.* Prominent lymphoplasmacytoid infiltration in an ordinary, predominantly transitional meningioma

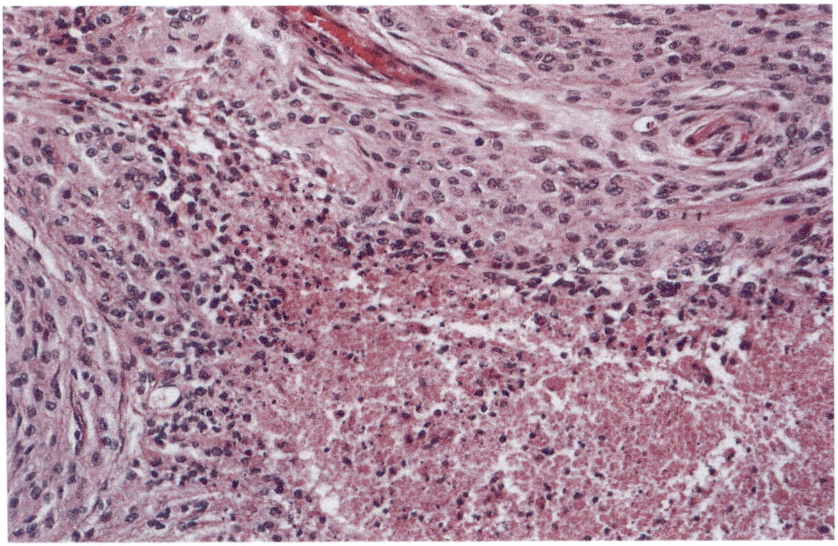

Fig.86. *Atypical meningioma* with increased mitotic activity and focal necrosis but preserved meningothelial differentiation

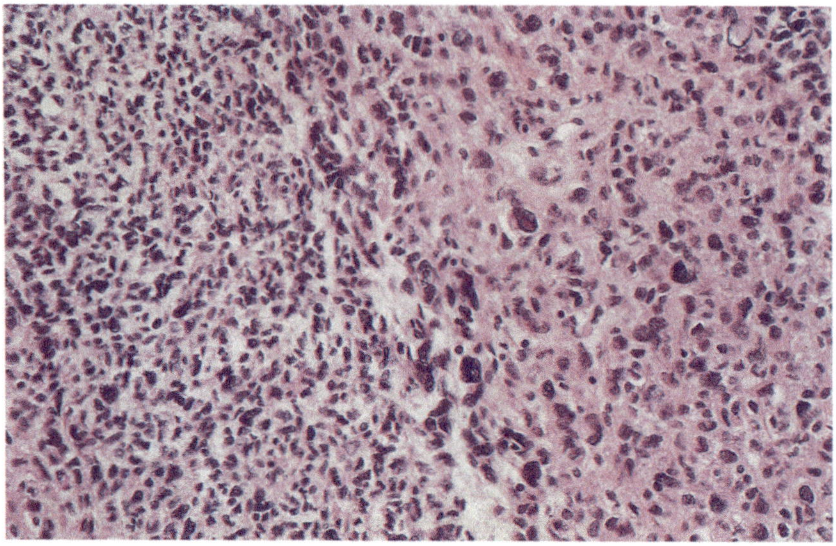

Fig. 87. *Atypical meningioma.* Marked nuclear atypia and extensive regressive small cell transition

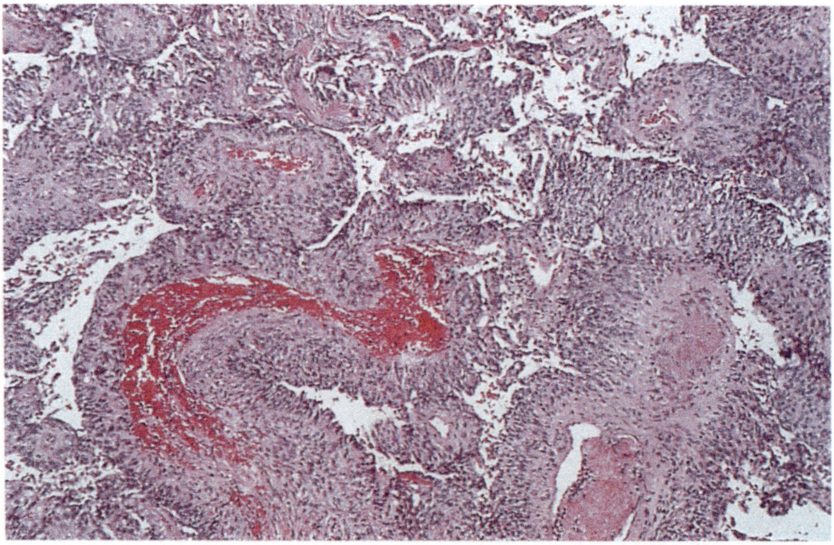

Fig. 88. *Papillary meningioma.* Highly cellular tumour forming papillary structures around vessel cores

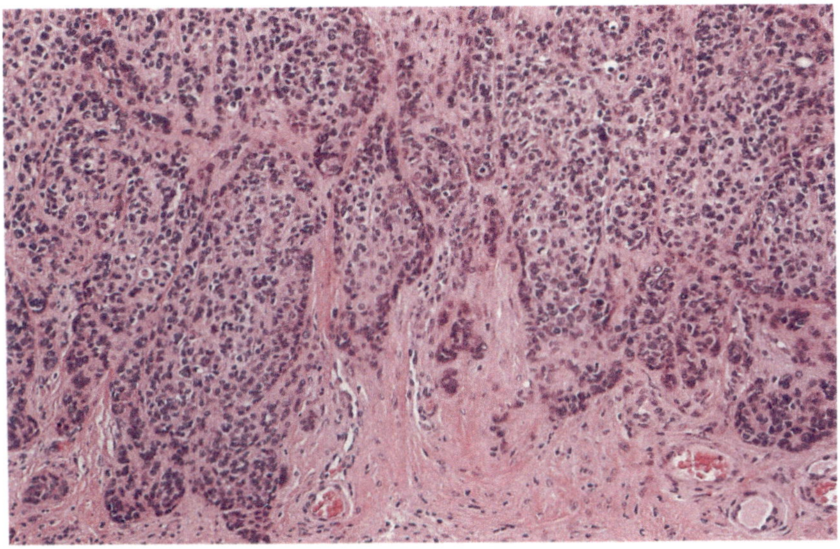

Fig.89. *Anaplastic (malignant) meningioma.* Highly cellular, patternless tumour with brisk mitotic activity and extensive invasion of the adjacent brain parenchyma

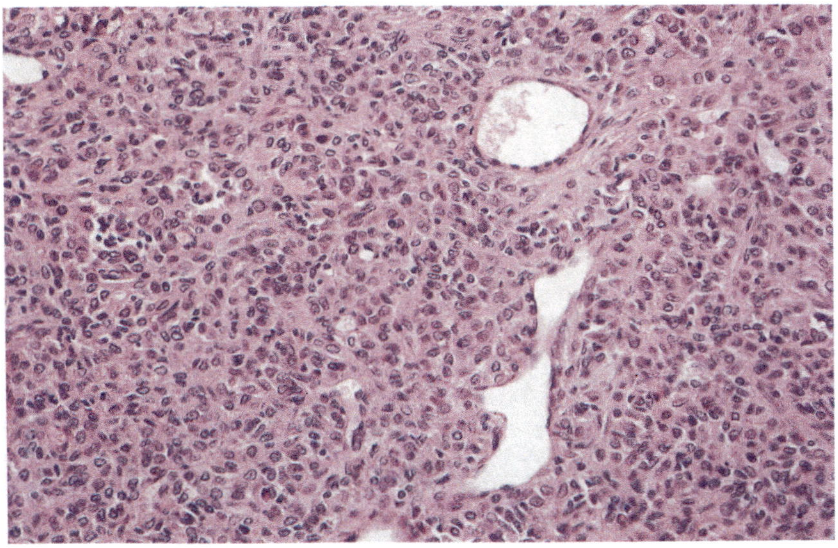

Fig.90. *Hemangiopericytoma.* Plump, polygonal tumour cells with increased mitotic activity in a dense fibrous stroma. Note the typical stag horn vasculature

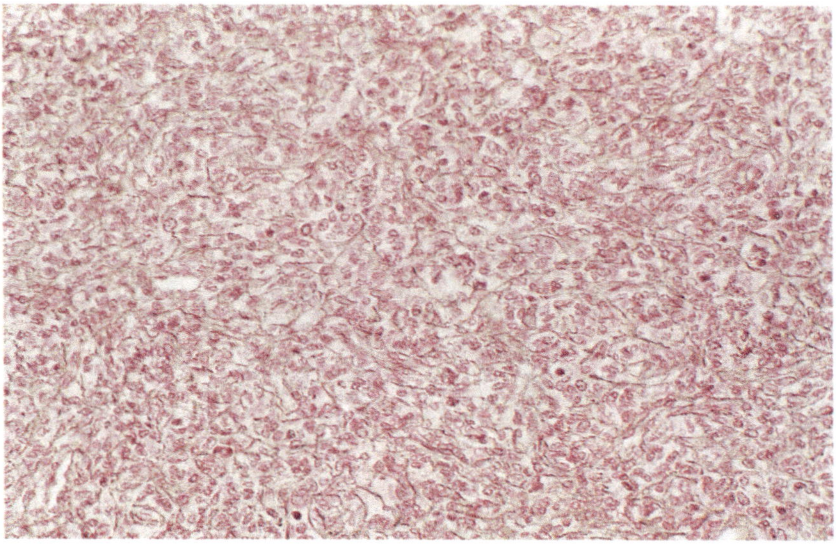

Fig. 91. *Hemangiopericytoma* with a typical dense, intercellular reticulin network

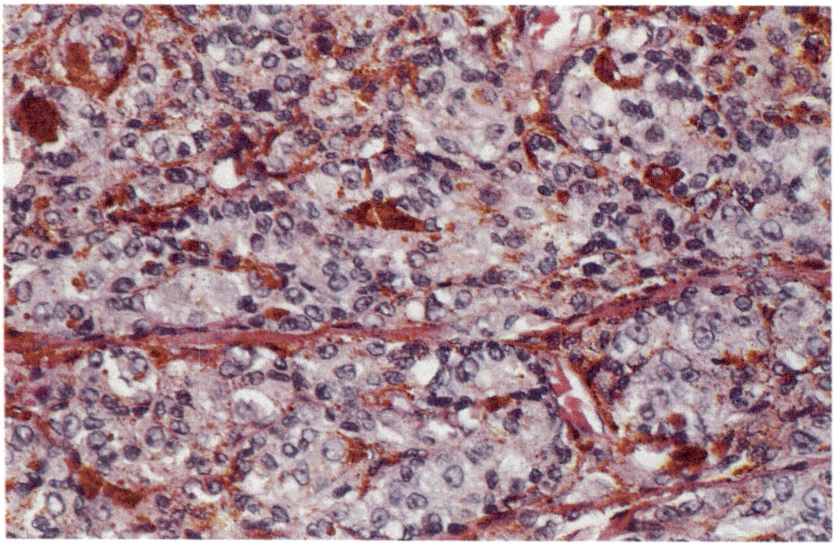

Fig. 92. *Melanocytoma*. Leptomeningeal tumour composed of sheet-like neoplastic melanocytes which often accumulate cytoplasmic melanin

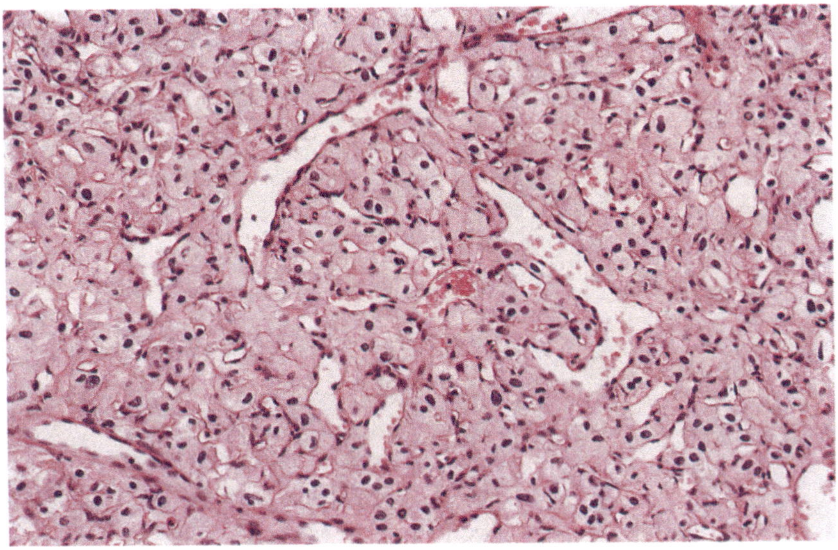

Fig.93. *Haemangioblastoma.* Tumour cells are distributed within a network of small and larger capillaries (reticular variant)

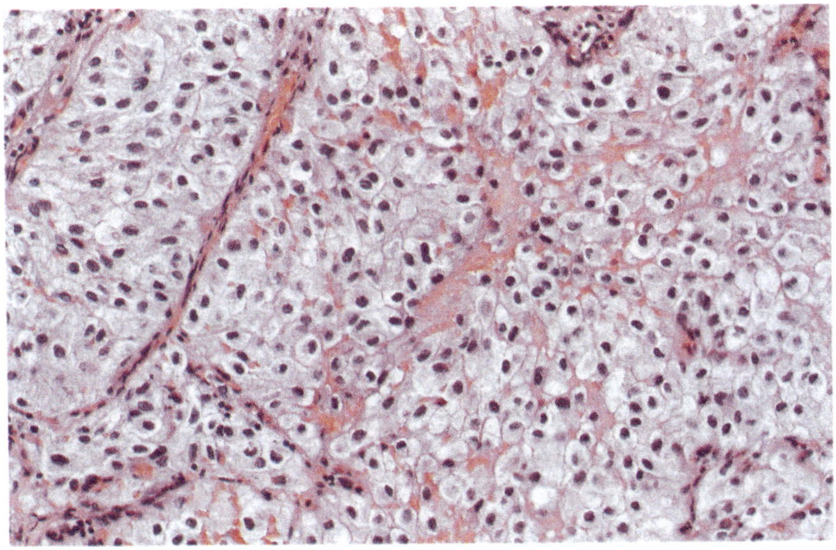

Fig.94. *Haemangioblastoma.* Densely packed tumour cells with clear, glycogen-rich cytoplasm (cellular variant) mimicking clear cell renal carcinoma

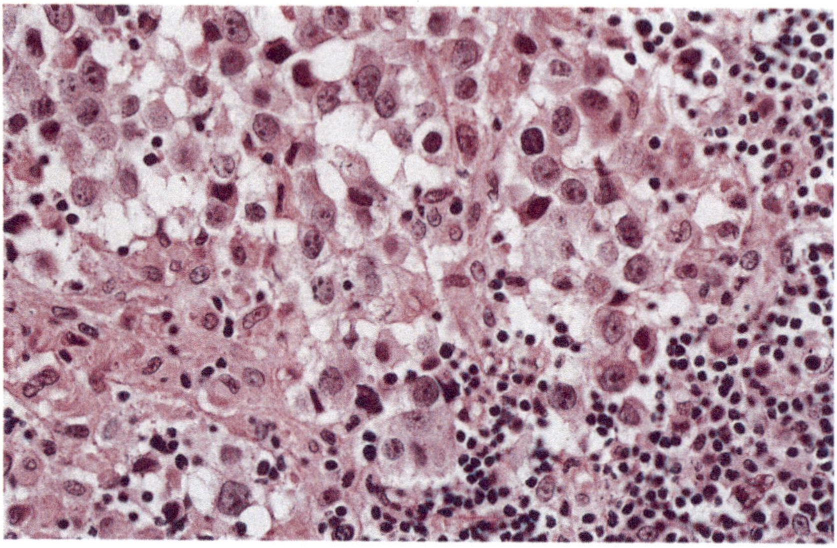

Fig.95. *Germinoma.* Tumor cells are uniformly large, with prominent nucleoli and clear, glycogen-rich cytoplasm. Note the typical lymphocytic infiltration

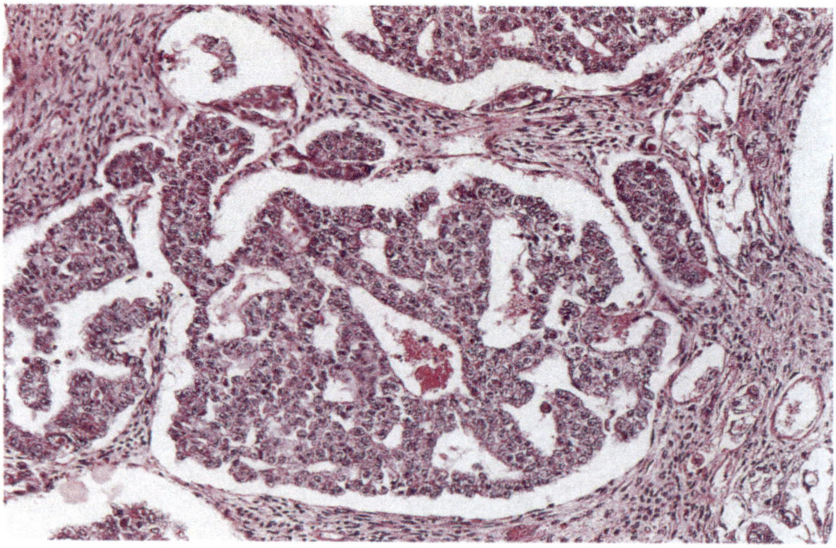

Fig.96. *Embryonal carcinoma.* Highly cellular, mitotically active primitive epithelia forming solid sheets and occasional poorly differentiated glands

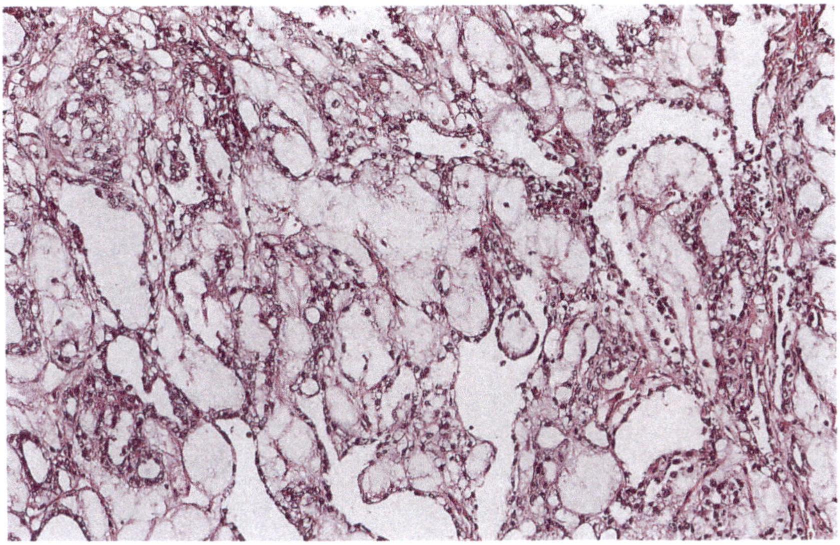

Fig. 97. *Yolk sac tumour (Endodermal sinus tumour).* Loosely textured cytologically malignant tumour cells in a reticular pattern

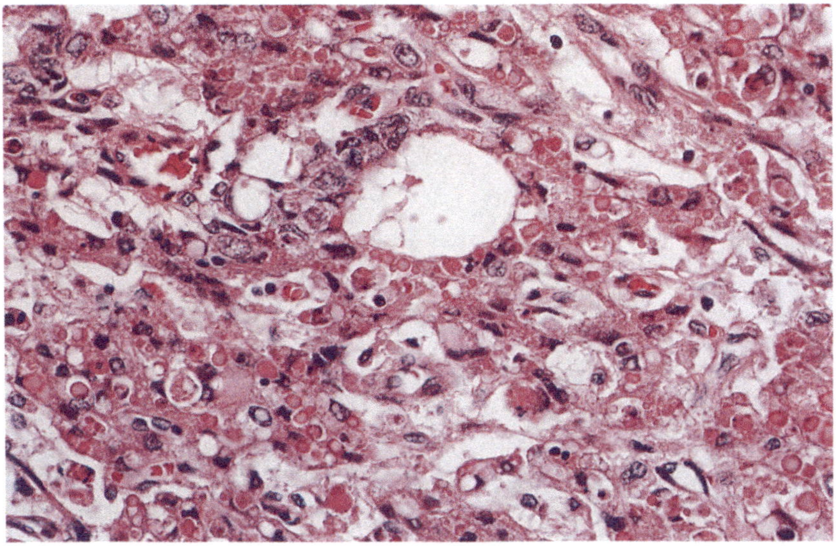

Fig. 98. *Yolk sac tumour (Endodermal sinus tumour).* Note the malignant epithelial cells and numerous hyaline globules characteristic of this tumour

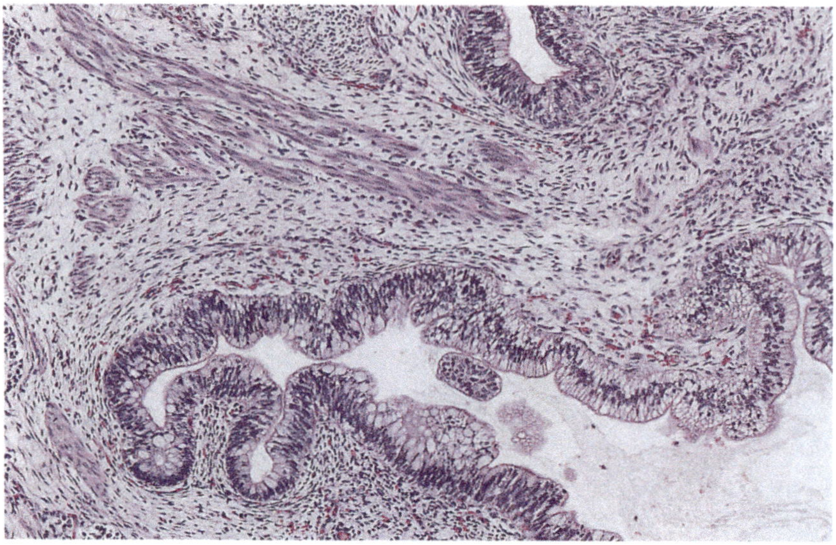

Fig. 99. *Immature teratoma* with primitive mesenchyme and glandular structures resembling fetal tissues

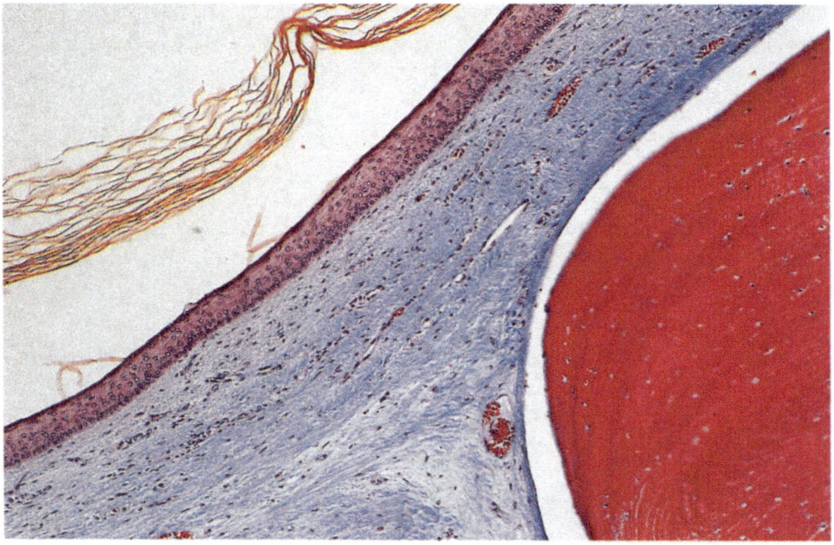

Fig. 100. *Mature teratoma* consisting of fully differentiated cartilage as well as squamous epithelium (trichrome stain)

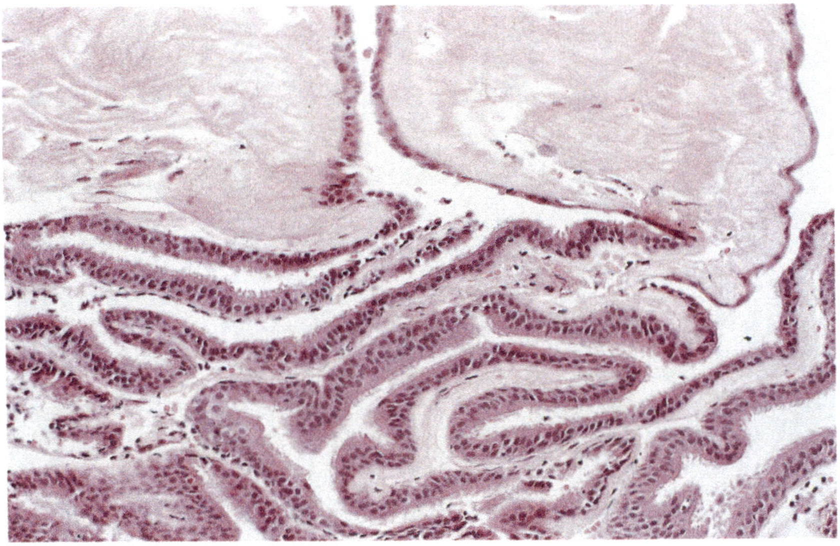

Fig. 101. *Rathke cleft cyst.* The lumen of the cyst is lined by a pseudostratified, ciliated epithelium which rests on a hyalinized stroma

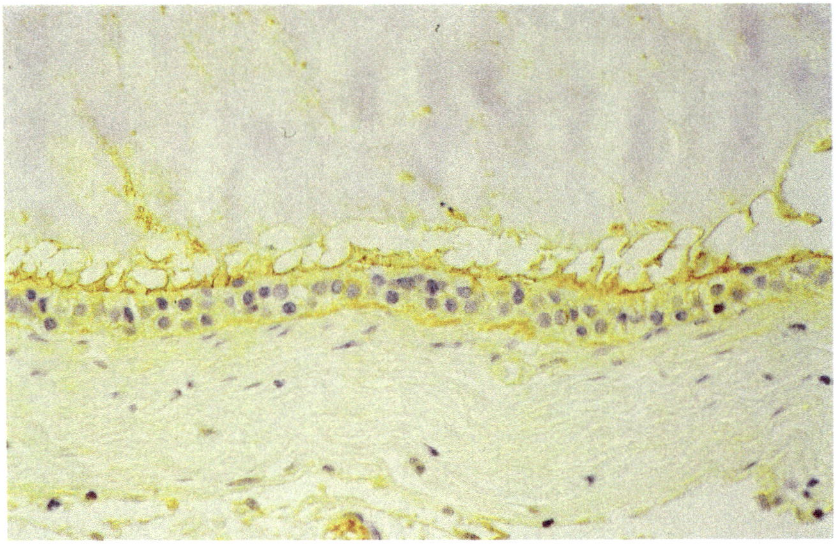

Fig. 102. *Colloid cyst of the third ventricle.* The lumen contains colloid-like material and is lined by ciliated, pseudostratified epithelium strongly expressing epithelial membrane antigen (EMA)

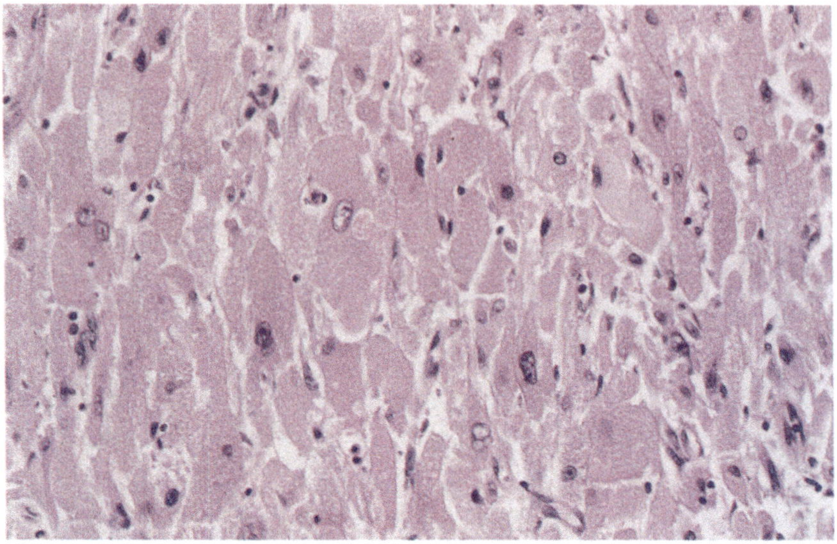

Fig. 103. *Granular cell tumour.* Large, polygonal cells with finely granular, eosinophilic cytoplasm

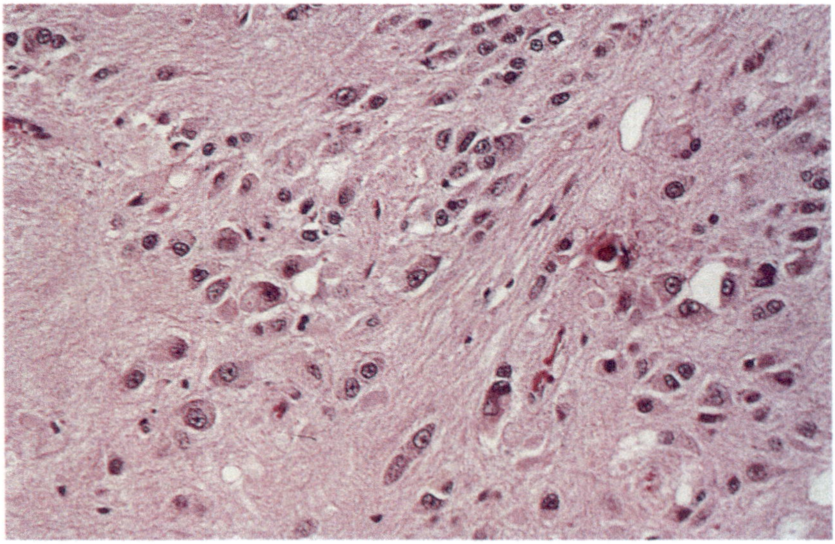

Fig. 104. *Hypothalamic neuronal hamartoma.* Clusters of mature, irregularly shaped neurons with an inconspicuous glial component

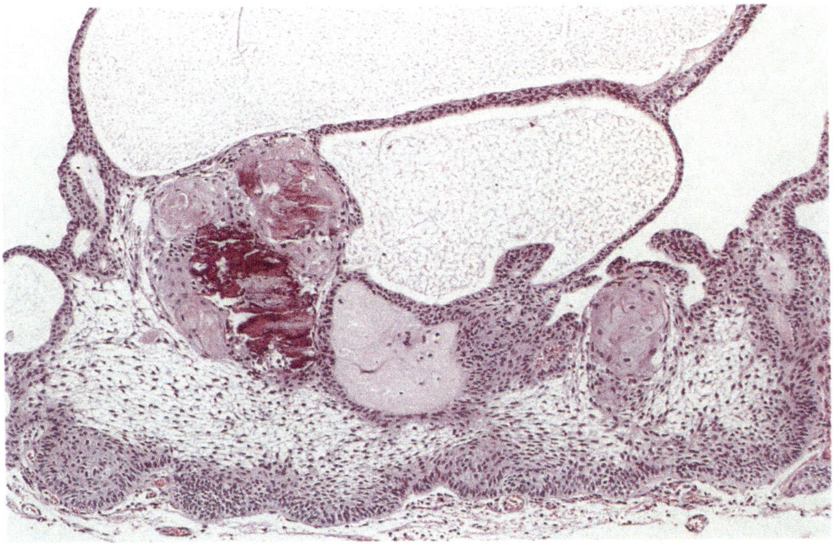

Fig. 105. *Adamantinomatous (classic) craniopharyngioma.* Squamous epithelial tumour cells forming large cysts. Note the peripheral palisading, and foci of keratin and calcification

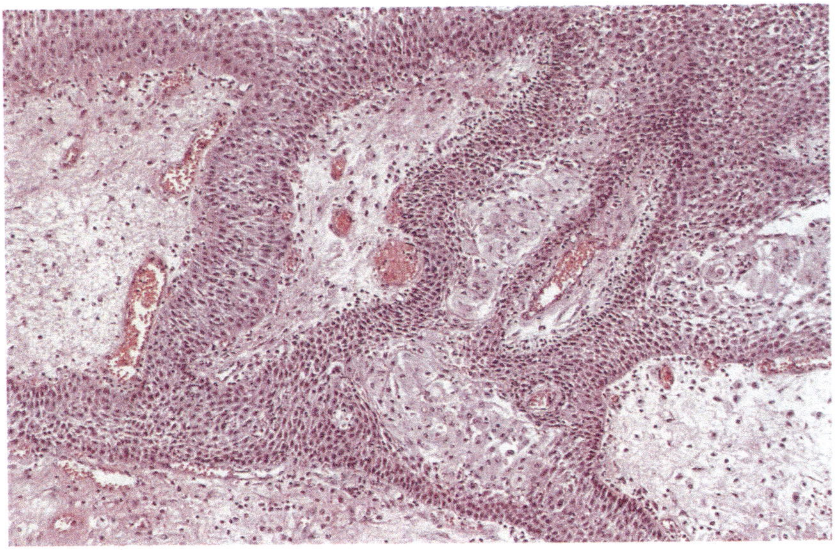

Fig. 106. *Papillary craniopharyngioma.* Well differentiated squamous epithelium forming pseudopapillary structures. Note the absence of keratinization and calcification

Subject Index

GPSR Compliance

The European Union's (EU) General Product Safety Regulation (GPSR) is a set of rules that requires consumer products to be safe and our obligations to ensure this.

If you have any concerns about our products, you can contact us on ProductSafety@springernature.com

In case Publisher is established outside the EU, the EU authorized representative is:

Springer Nature Customer Service Center GmbH
Europaplatz 3
69115 Heidelberg, Germany

Batch number: 10704763

Printed by Printforce, the Netherlands